Practical Handbook of Echocardiography

Companion Website

http://booksupport.wiley.com

This books is accompanied by a website with:
- A database of 366 video clips
- Video clips are all referenced in the text where you see this symbol:

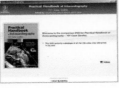
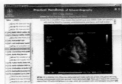
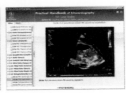

Practical Handbook of Echocardiography

101 Case Studies

Edited by

Jing Ping Sun, MD

Associate Professor of Medicine
Emory University School of Medicine
Emory University Hospital Midtown
Atlanta, GA
USA

Joel M. Felner, MD

Associate Dean (Clinical Education)
Professor of Medicine
Emory University School of Medicine
Director of Echocardiography
Grady Memorial Hospital
Emory University School of Medicine
Atlanta, GA
USA

John D. Merlino, MD

Assistant Professor
Emory University School of Medicine
Director of Echocardiography Laboratory
Emory University Hospital Midtown
Atlanta, GA
USA

WILEY-BLACKWELL

A John Wiley & Sons, Ltd., Publication

Library of Congress Cataloging-in-Publication Data
Practical handbook of echocardiography/edited by Jing Ping Sun, Joel M. Felner, John D. Merlino.
   p. ; cm.
   Includes bibliographical references and index.
   ISBN 978-1-4051-9556-0 (pbk. : alk. paper)   1. Echocardiography–Handbooks, manuals, etc.
I. Sun, Jingping.   II. Felner, Joel M., 1942-   III. Merlino, John D.
   [DNLM: 1. Echocardiography–methods.   2. Cardiovascular Diseases–ultrasonography. WG
141.5.E2 P89403 2010]
   RC683.5.U5P717 2010
   616.1′207543–dc22
                                                                           2010015119

ISBN: 9781405195560

A catalogue record for this book is available from the British Library.

Set in 9.25/11.5pt Minion by Aptara® Inc., New Delhi, India

1   2010

Contents

Part 9   Infective Disease

Companion Website	http://booksupport.wiley.com

This books is accompanied by a website with:
- A database of 366 video clips
- Video clips are all referenced in the text where you see this symbol: 👁

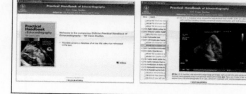
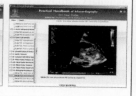

List of Contributors

Vasilus Babaliaros, MD
Assistant Professor
Emory University School of Medicine;
Emory University Hospital Midtown
Atlanta, GA
USA

Robert C. Bahler, MD
Professor of Medicine
Case Western University;
Staff Physician
Heart and Vascular Center
MetroHealth Medical Center
Cleveland, OH
USA

Ambareesh Bajpai, MD
Cardiology Fellow
Emory University School of Medicine
Emory University Hospital Midtown
Atlanta, GA
USA

Patrick E. BeDell, RDCS
Clinical Directory
Xinjiang Medical School
Urumqi
China

Leilei Cheng, MD
Lecturer in Cardiology
Fudan University;
Attending Doctor
Echocardiography Laboratory
Shanghai Cardiovascular Diseases Institute
Zhongshan Hospital
Fudan University
Shanghai
China

Seth Clemens, MD
Assistant professor
Emory University School of Medicine
Emory University Hospital Midtown
Atlanta, GA
USA

Yan Deng, MD
Associate Chief Physician
Southwest Jiaotong University;
Staff Physician
Department of Cardiovascular Ultrasound & Non Invasive Cardiology
Sichuan Academy of Medical Sciences
Sichuan Provincial People's Hospital
Chengdu
China

Gui Chun Ding, MD
Technician of Sonography
The Second Military Medical University
Shanghai;
The General Hospital of Beijing Military Command of PLA
Beijing
China

Joel M. Felner, MD
Associate Dean (Clinical Education)
Professor of Medicine
Emory University School of Medicine;
Director of Echocardiography
Grady Memorial Hospital
Emory University School of Medicine
Atlanta, GA
USA

LuYue Gai, MD
Department of Cardiology
General Hospital of PLA
Beijing
China

Erin Galbraith, MD
Cardiovascular Disease Fellow
Emory University School of Medicine
Emory University Hospital Midtown
Atlanta, GA
USA

Yunhua Gao, MD
Professor in Medicine
The Third Military Medical University;
Director, Department of Ultrasound
XinQiao Hospital
ChongQing
China

Lin He, MD
Physician in charge of Cardiology
Huazhong University of Science and Technology;
Staff Physician
Department of Ultrasonography
Union Hospital of Hust
Wuhan, Hubei
China

Yuhai Ho, MD
Department of Ultrasound
Beijing Anzhen Hospital
Capital Medical University
Beijing
China

Ming-Jui Hung, MD
Associate Professor of Medicine
Chang Gung University College of Medicine;
Staff Physician
Adult Cardiology
Chang Gung Memorial Hospital at Keelung
Keelung
Taiwan

Shuang Li, MD
Attending Physician
Southwest Jiaotong University;
Staff Physician
Department of Cardiovascular Ultrasound Non Invasive Medicine
Sichuan Academy of Medical Sciences
Sichuan Provincial People's Hospital
Chengdu, Sichuan
China

Zhi An Li, MD
Director of Department of Ultrasound
Beijing Anzhen Hospital
Capital Medical University
Beijing
China

Wen Xu Liu, MD
Department of Ultrasound
Beijing Anzhen Hospital
Capital Medical University
Beijing
China

Xiaofang Lu, MD
Huazhong University of Science and Technology
Union Hospital of HUST
Wuhan, Hubei
China

John D. Merlino, MD
Assistant Professor
Emory University School of Medicine;
Director of Echocardiography Laboratory
Emory University Hospital Midtown
Atlanta, GA
USA

Yuming Mu, MD
Director
Department of Ultrasound
XinJiang Medical School
Urumqi
China

Robert D. O'Donnell Jr., MD
Assistant Professor of Cardiology
Emory University School of Medicine;
Director
Cardiac MRI & CTA
Emory University Hospital Midtown
Atlanta, GA
USA

Pin Qian, MD
Lecturer in Ultrasonography
The Third Military Medical University;
Staff Physician
Department of Ultrasound
XinQiao Hospital
Chonhqing
China

Alicia N. Rangosch RDCS, RUT
Echo Technician
Emory University School of Medicine
Emory University Hospital Midtown
Atlanta, GA
USA

Xianhong Shu, MD
Director
Department of Ultrasound
Shanghai Cardiovascular Diseases Institute
Zhongshan Hospital
Fudan University
China

Dan Sorescu, MD, FACC
Cardiologist
Emory University School of Medicine;
Emory University Hospital Midtown
Atlanta, GA
USA

William J. Stewart, MD
The Cleveland Clinic Foundation
Cleveland, OH
USA

Angela K. Sullivan CCT, RCS
Emory University School of Medicine;
Emory University Hospital Midtown
Atlanta, GA
USA

Jing Ping Sun, MD
Associate Professor of Medicine
Emory University School of Medicine;
Emory University Hospital Midtown
Atlanta, GA
USA

Hong Tang, MD
Professor of Cardiology
Sichuan University
Chengdu, Sichuan
China

James D. Thomas, MD
Professor of Medicine
Director of Cardiovascular Image
The Cleveland Clinic Foundation
Cleveland, OH
USA

Jian Hua Wang, PhD
Professor of Cardiology
The Second Military Medical University
Shanghai;
Director
Echocardiography Department
The General Hospital of Beijing Military Command of PLA
Beijing
China

Shan Wang, MD
Attending Physician
Southwest Jiaotong University;
Staff Physician
Department of Cardiovascular Ultrasound Non Invasive Medicine
Sichuan Academy of Medical Sciences
Sichuan Provincial People's Hospital
Chengdu, Sichuan
China

Xin-Fang Wang, MD
Professor of Cardiology
Huazhong University of Science and Technology;
Professor of Echo Lab
Union Hospital of HUST
Wuhan, Hubei
China

Zheng-Yang Wang, MD
Attending Physician
Southwest Jiaotong University;
Staff Physician
Department of Cardiovascular Ultrasound Non Invasive Medicine
Sichuan Academy of Medical Sciences
Sichuan Provincial People's Hospital
Chengdu, Sichuan
China

Byron R. Williams Jr., MD
Martha West Looney Professor of Medicine
Emory University School of Medicine;
Chief of Internal Medicine
Emory University Hospital Midtown
Atlanta, GA
USA

Ming Xing Xie, MD, PhD
Professor of Cardiology
Huazhong University of Science and Technology;
Director of Echocardiography
Lab of Union Hospital
Union Hospital of HUST
Wuhan, Hubei
China

Yali Xu, MD
Lecturer in Ultrasonography
The Third Military Medical University;
Staff Physician
Department of Ultrasound
XinQiao Hospital
ChongQing
China

Shawn X. Yang, MD, PhD
Staff Physician
Memorial Hermann Southwest Medical Center
Houston, TX
USA

Xing Sheng Yang, MD, PhD
Emory University School of Medicine
Emory University Hospital Midtown
Atlanta, GA
USA

Li-xue Yin, MD
Professor of Medicine
Southwest Jiaotong University;
Director
Department of Cardiovascular Ultrasound & Non Invasive Cardiology
Chief Physician
Cardiology, Sichuan Academy of Medical Sciences
Sichuan Provincial People's Hospital
Chengdu, Sichuan
China

Dale Yoo, MD
Cardiac Electrophysiology Fellow
Emory University School of Medicine;
Housestaff
Cardiac Electrophysiology
Emory University Hospital
Atlanta, GA
USA

Yang Yu, MD
Attending Physician
Southwest Jiaotong University;
Staff Physician
Department of Cardiovascular Ultrasound & Non Invasive Cardiology
Sichuan Academy of Medical Sciences
Sichuan Provincial People's Hospital
Chengdu, Sichuan
China

Xiao Juan Zhang, MD
Pediatrician
Department of Cardiology
General Hospital of PLA
Beijing
China

Guang Zhi, MD
Department of Cardiology
General Hospital of PLA
Beijing
China

Ming-liang Zuo, MD
Attending Physician
Southwest Jiaotong University;
Staff Physician
Department of Cardiovascular Ultrasound Non Invasive Medicine
Sichuan Academy of Medical Sciences
Sichuan Provincial People's Hospital
Chengdu, Sichuan
China

Preface

The field of echocardiography is of great importance to the care of patients with a problem involving the cardiovascular system. Virtually, all patients with suspected or known cardiovascular diseases undergo echocardiographic analysis as part of their evaluation. The dramatic increase in the application and understanding of echocardiography has made echocardiography one of the most requested imaging modalities in the twenty-first century. In the past two decades there has been extensive development in the field with the increased use of transesophageal and three-dimensional echocardiography. As a consequence of this rapid development it has been difficult for practicing physicians to understand all of the many uses and innovations in this field.

This volume was created in response to these developments. Its goal is to present excellent illustrations of both common and unusual echocardiograms using a case-based format. It is not meant to be a general textbook of echocardiography. We purposely omitted a detailed discussion of the procedure and the advantages and disadvantages of the technique. These topics are well discussed in other echocardiographic books.

The idea of the book originated from the need to provide excellent illustrations, using both still and real-time images. We asked many echocardiographic leaders and a large number of the cardiology fellows at Emory University School of Medicine what they thought was lacking in the available literature. It is apparent that a case-based echocardiographic book is necessary and the need for well-described and detailed illustrations of unusual cases and unusual presentations of common cases is also needed. We, therefore, chose 101 cases out of more than 5000 cases we perused to illustrate common and uncommon conditions. The book is organized in 12 sections covering all of the cardiovascular lesions that are encountered daily. The sections on trauma and masses cover material that is not easily found in the literature. In planning this book, several guiding principles were followed. The editors have expertise in the entire gamut of echocardiography. All of the chapters were chosen so that each area of cardiology is well represented. Both still images and real-time studies were included because they could be labeled easily and illustrate clearly important echocardiographic principles. We included some common conditions, e.g., mitral stenosis and some unusual cases, e.g., of an unroofed coronary sinus atrial septal defect. Each illustration is labeled in detail with the modality and transducer position identified. The case presentation is followed by a short discussion, including treatment, and pertinent references. In addition to the basic interpretation, special emphasis is given to occult findings. It is hoped that the reader will find these illustrations both instructive and beguiling. Because of the restriction on the number of cases and the number of pages permitted, every illustration of an abnormality and further detail of the cases were curtailed. We did include a short discussion of the case and pertinent references.

It is our hope that cardiologists, in private practice and in academic medical centers, and physicians in training will benefit from the many illustrations and overall design of this book. It provides a rapid guide and reference to a broad spectrum of echocardiographic images and the case-based format should make it particularly valuable to physicians, house officers, and technicians.

We wish to acknowledge with great appreciation the efforts of all of the technicians at Emory University School of Medicine, and in particular, Kay Rubenstein-Felner, for her reading of the entire manuscript and correcting any errors in syntax and grammar. In addition, we wish to thank all of the physicians who have contributed the cases.

Jing Ping Sun, Joel M. Felner, John D. Merlino

Abbreviations

2D, two-dimensional echocardiography
A2-ch, apical 2-chamber
A3-ch, apical 3-chamber
A4-ch, apical 4-chamber
A5-ch, apical 5-chamber
AAO, ascending aorta
ABDA, abdomen aorta
ABS, apical ballooning syndrome
AF, atrial fibrillation
AICD, automatic implantable cardioverter defibrillator
AMIS, aneurysm of the membranous interventricular septum
AMI, acute myocardial infarction
AO, aorta
AR, aortic regurgitation
AS, aortic valve stenosis
ASA, atrial septal aneurysm
ASD, atrial septal defect
AV, aortic valve
BP, blood pressure
CAD, coronary artery disease
CHF, congestive heart failure
CP, constrictive pericarditis
CS, coronary sinus
CRT, cardiac resynchronization therapy
CT, computed tomography
DAO, descending aorta
DCRV, double-chambered right ventricle
DFSS, discrete fixed fibromuscular subaortic stenosis
DMSS, discrete fixed membranous subaortic stenosis
ECG, electrocardiogram
EF, ejection fraction
EKG, electrocardiogram
HCM, hypertrophic cardiomyopathy
HF, heart failure
HR, heart rate
IAA, interrupted aortic arch
IAS, interatrial septum
ICMV, isolated cleft mitral valve

ICU, intensive care unit
IE, infectious endocarditis
IMH, aortic intramural hematoma
IVC, inferior vena cava
IVS, interventricular septum
LAA, left atrial appendage
LAD, left anterior descending
LPA, left pulmonary artery
LUPV, left upper pulmonary vein
LA, left atrium
LV, left ventricle
LVD, left ventricular diverticulum/diverticula
LVH, left ventricular hypertrophy
LVOT, left ventricular outflow tract
M-mode, time motion mode
MCA, main coronary artery
MI, myocardial infarction
MR, mitral regurgitation
MRI, magnetic resonance imaging
MS, mitral valve stenosis
MV, mitral valve
MVA, mitral valve area
MVP, mitral valve prolapse
PA, pulmonary artery
PAU, penetrating atheromatous ulcer
PDA, patent duct artery
PEff, pericardial effusion
PFO, patent foramen ovale
PLA, parasternal long axis
PlEff, pleural effusion
PSA, parasternal short-axis
PV, pulmonic valve
PVT, prosthetic valve thrombosis
RA, right atrium
RCA, right coronary artery
RCM, restrictive cardiomyopathy
RPA, right pulmonary artery
RUPV, right upper pulmonary vein
RV, right ventricle
RVOT, right ventricular outflow tract
SAM, systolic anterior motion
SBP, systolic blood pressure
SC, subcostal
SSN, suprasternal notch
SV, stroke volume
SVC, superior vena cava
TOF, tetralogy of Fallot
TR, tricuspid regurgitation

TSE, turbo spin echo
TSS, tunnel subaortic stenosis
TV, tricuspid valve
UCSD, unroofed coronary sinus defect
URCS, unroofed coronary sinus
VSD, ventricular septal defect
VTI, velocity time integral

Part 1
Aortic Diseases

1 Spontaneous Ruptured Aneurysm of the Sinus of Valsalva

Jing Ping Sun[1], Xing Sheng Yang[1] & James D. Thomas[2]

[1] Emory University School of Medicine; Emory University Hospital Midtown, Atlanta, GA, USA
[2] The Cleveland Clinic Foundation, Cleveland, OH, USA

History

Case 1: A 30-year-old female had no symptom. Cardiology examination revealed a grade 4/6 diastolic heart murmur at the left sternal edge.

Transthoracic echocardiography (TTE): An aneurysm of the right sinus of Valsalva was well seen in the parasternal short-axis (PSA) view. The aneurysm was ruptured into right ventricle (RV) as demonstrated by color Doppler (Figure 1.1 and Videoclip 1.1).

Case 2: A 40-year-old male had the onset of a new heart murmur. Auscultation revealed grades 3/6 systolic and 3/6 diastolic murmurs best heard at the right sternal border.

Echocardiogram revealed that left ventricle (LV) and RV were normal in size and systolic function. A PSA view with color Doppler shows a ruptured aneurysm of the noncoronary sinus of Valsalva and the high-velocity flow through the ruptured noncoronary sinus aneurysm into right atrium (RA; Figure 1.2 and Videoclip 1.2).

Discussion

A ruptured aneurysm of aortic sinus is a major cardiovascular event that demands prompt diagnosis and treatment. Most aortic sinuses of Valsalva aneurysms are congenital or are associated with an infectious process such as endocarditis or syphilis. In our two cases, the patient presented at 30 and 40 years of age. The anatomical positions of the coronary sinus and the aortic valve are normal, and predisposing infection is absent, which suggests a possible spontaneous rupture of congenital coronary sinus aneurysms.

The right sinus of Valsalva is the most common site of aortic sinus aneurysmal dilatation, followed by the noncoronary sinus. After rupture, a fistulous tract is formed, frequently with the RV in the former instance and with the RA in the latter [1]. Uncommonly, rupture into the pulmonary artery may occur [2]. Our patients had a ruptured right and noncoronary

Practical Handbook of Echocardiography 1st edition. Edited by Jing Ping Sun, Joel Felner and John Merlino. © 2010 Blackwell Publishing Ltd.

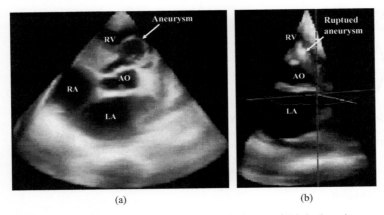

Figure 1.1. (a) Parasternal short-axis view shows the right sinus of Valsalva (arrow). (b) Parasternal short-axis view with color Doppler shows the high-velocity flow through the ruptured sinus aneurysm into right ventricle in case 1. AO, aorta; LA, left atrium; RA, right atrium; RV, right ventricle.

sinus of Valsalva and a fistula to the RV in case 1 and to the RA in case 2. At presentation, they had the onset of a new murmur and had no symptoms, which suggests that these events happened recently.

TTE can lead to an accurate diagnosis in most of these patients and transesophageal echocardiography may be useful when TTE is inconclusive. The natural history of asymptomatic aneurysm of an aortic sinus is unclear, and variant cases—with rapid clinical deterioration or many years of stabilization—have been described [1]. However, once symptoms develop or rupture occurs, urgent intervention is recommended. Open-heart correction of the aneurysm and fistula, with or

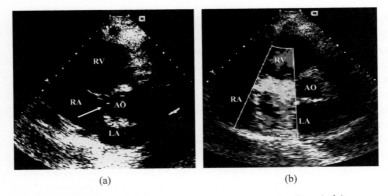

Figure 1.2. (a) Parasternal short-axis view shows ruptured aneurysm (arrow) of the noncoronary sinus of Valsalva. (b) Parasternal short-axis view with color Doppler illustrates the high-velocity flow through the ruptured noncoronary sinus aneurysm into right atrium in case 2. AO, aorta; LA, left atrium; RA, right atrium; RV, right ventricle.

without aortic valve replacement, carries a low operative risk and traditionally has been the choice of treatment [1]. A novel percutaneous closure technique has brought hope of a less invasive method to correct such condition [3]. Our patient underwent a traditional operation and recovered completely.

References

1. Takach TJ, Reul GJ, Duncan JM, *et al.* Sinus of Valsalva aneurysm or fistula: management and outcome. *Ann Thorac Surg* 1999;68:1573–7.
2. Luckraz H, Naik M, Jenkins G, Youhana A. Repair of a sinus of Valsalva aneurysm that had ruptured into the pulmonary artery. *J Thorac Cardiovasc Surg* 2004;127:1823–5.
3. Fedson S, Jolly N, Lang RM, Hijazi ZM. Percutaneous closure of a ruptured sinus of Valsalva aneurysm using the Amplatzer Duct Occluder. *Catheter Cardiovasc Interv* 2003;58:406–11.

2 Sinus of Valsalva Aneurysms

Jing Ping Sun, Xing Sheng Yang & John D. Merlino
Emory University School of Medicine; Emory University Hospital Midtown, Atlanta, GA, USA

History

A 50-year-old female complains of dyspnea on exertion.

Physical Examination

Heart rate was 69 bpm and a 2/6 systolic murmur was noted.

Echocardiography

Transthoracic echocardiography: The left ventricle and the right ventricle were normal in size and in systolic function. Left atrium and right atrium were normal in size. Two large aneurysms involving the noncoronary and right coronary cusps with partial obstruction of the right ventricular outflow tract were noted (Figure 2.1).

Transesophageal echocardiographic short-axis view shows two huge aneurysms of right and noncoronary sinuses with spontaneous contrast (Videoclip 2.1).

Discussion

Aneurysms of the sinus of Valsalva are usually diagnosed as an incidental finding or after an acute rupture into an adjacent cardiac structure. Before rupture, aneurysms of the sinus of Valsalva may present with conduction-system abnormalities attributable to erosion into the interventricular septum. Thromboembolism originating in the aneurysm sac, which is attributable to coronary compression [1].

Sawyers *et al.* demonstrated a mean survival period of 4 years in patients with untreated ruptured sinuses of Valsalva aneurysms; early surgical intervention is recommended [2]. The optimal management of an asymptomatic, nonruptured aneurysm is less clear because of the absence of a precise natural history [3]. Improvements in surgical technique in the past 15 years have resulted in low complication rates with no early mortality (0%) and low morbidity (4%) [3].

Practical Handbook of Echocardiography 1st edition. Edited by Jing Ping Sun, Joel Felner and John Merlino. © 2010 Blackwell Publishing Ltd.

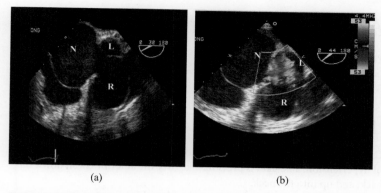

(a)   (b)

Figure 2.1. Transesophageal echocardiography: The trileaflet aortic valve with two huge aneurysms of right and noncoronary sinuses is well seen during diastole (a) and systole with color flow (b). L, left coronary sinus; N, noncoronary sinus; R, right coronary sinus.

Our case had two large aneurysms that involved right and noncoronary sinuses, which is rare. Because of the unusually large size of the aneurysms, this patient underwent aortic root replacement with left coronary implantation and right coronary artery bypass without complication.

References

1. Feldman DN, Roman MJ. Aneurysms of the sinuses of Valsalva. *Cardiology* 2006;106:73–81.
2. Sawyers JL, Adams JE, Scott HW Jr. Surgical treatment for aneurysms of the aortic sinuses with aorticoatrial fistula. *Surgery* 1957;41:26–42.
3. Moustafa S, Mookadam F, Cooper L, *et al.* Sinus of Valsalva aneurysms—47 years of a single center experience and systematic overview of published reports. *Am J Cardiol* 2007;99:1159–64.

3 Aortic Dissection

Xing Sheng Yang & Jing Ping Sun

Emory University School of Medicine; Emory University Hospital Midtown, Atlanta, GA, USA

History

Case 1: A 60-year-old female is admitted with chest pain. She has a history of hypertension. The pain is pressure-like over the anterior chest, down the back, and up into the neck.

    Case 2: A 40-year-old male presented with sudden onset of severe chest pain with diaphoresis and shortness of breath.

Physical Examination

Case 1: Blood pressure (BP) was 180/100 mmHg, pulse rate was 102/minute, and respiration rate was 30/minute. All other physical findings were unremarkable.

    Case 2: BP was 240/120 mmHg, heart rate was 82/minute and regular. Auscultation: 2/6 mid-systolic murmur.

Laboratory

Case 1: Electrocardiogram showed left ventricle hypertrophy (LVH). Chest X-ray revealed a widening in the aortic knob and the lateral margin of the ascending aorta. Computed tomography revealed an aortic dissection extending from the aortic root to descending aorta (DAO).

    Echocardiography revealed (1) concentric LVH; (2) ejection fraction 55%; and (3) small pericardial effusion. Linear echodensities within the lumen of the aortic root parallel to the wall of the aorta compatible with an intimal flap were seen (Videoclip 3.1). There was moderate to severe aortic regurgitation (AR). The aortic annulus and root were dilated. Transesophageal echocardiography (TEE): parasetenal long-axis view shows dilated aortic root with intimal flap and short-axis view shows clot, true, and false lumen (Figure 3.1).

    Case 2: chest X-ray showed mild cardiomegaly. Magnetic resonance imaging (MRI) showed a type B aortic dissection tracking into abdominal aorta (Videoclip 3.2a).

    Echocardiography: the aortic arch from supersternal notch showed dilated ascending aorta (AAO) with intimal flap and DAO with true and false lumina (Figure 3.2, Videoclip 3.2d).

Practical Handbook of Echocardiography 1st edition. Edited by Jing Ping Sun, Joel Felner and John Merlino. © 2010 Blackwell Publishing Ltd.

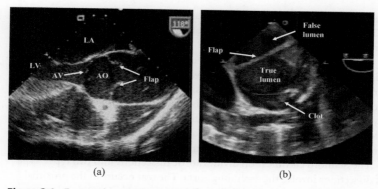

(a)   (b)

Figure 3.1. Transesophageal echocardiography: (a) parasetenal long-axis view shows dilated aortic root with intimal flap (arrow). (b) Basal short-axis view shows clot, true, and false lumen. AO, aorta; AV, aortic valve; LA, left atrium; LV, left ventricle.

Abdominal aortic dissection with small true and large false lumens were seen. TEE long-axis view indicated the color flows from true lumen into false lumen through intimal flap (Videoclip 3.2).

The echocardiographic characteristics of aortic dissection from other cases are shown in Videoclip 3.3.

Discussion

Aortic dissection is a common fatal disorder in which the inner layer of the aortic wall tears because the artery's wall deteriorates. Most cases are associated with hypertension.

Conventional transthoracic echocardiography (TTE) is useful in ascending aortic dissections and has limited diagnostic value in the

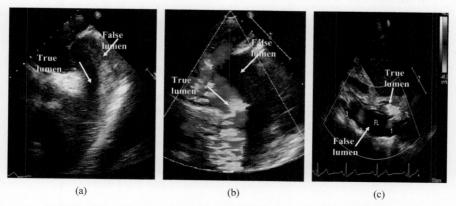

(a)   (b)   (c)

Figure 3.2. Transthoracic echocardiography: (a) the aortic arch from supersternal notch shows dilated ascending aorta with intimal flap, and descending aorta with true and false lumina (arrows). (b) The true and false lumina (arrows) are well seen in the same aortic arch with color Doppler. (c) Transsurface image shows an abdominal aortic dissection with small true and large false lumens; there are communications between true and false lumina.

evaluation of the thoracic aorta. Combined the information of multiple TTE views and TEE for the diagnosis of acute aortic dissection is important.

The echocardiographic characteristics in the diagnosis of aortic dissection are (1) the presence of two vascular lumens separated by an undulating intimal flap; (2) the entry site of the dissection is commonly defined as a tear of the dissected membrane with blood flow demonstrated by color Doppler between the two aortic lumina; and (3) the direction of blood flow across the entry tear of the aortic dissection follows the pressure gradient between the false and true lumina.

The Stanford classification divides aortic dissections into two types: type A dissections involve the ascending aorta. The tear occurs in the proximal AAO and can extend into DAO. Type B is originated in DAO distal to the left subclavian artery and extends mostly above the diaphragm; they may track into abdominal aorta [1].

In case 1, the tear arose proximal to the left subclavian artery and extended proximally to involve the ascending aorta; this aortic dissection is classified as type A. Aortic regurgitation and pericardial effusion, as seen in our patient, are findings frequently associated with proximal aortic dissections.

Magnetic resonance and echocardiographic images demonstrated the aortic dissection tracking into abdominal aorta in case 2, which should belong to aortic dissection type B.

Erosion of the internal elastic membrane that lies beneath an inflammatory atherosclerotic plaque may allow luminal blood to burrow into the aortic media and thus lead to the formation of a penetrating aortic ulcer (Videoclip 3.3d).

In acute type A dissections immediate surgery is generally recommended, unless comorbidities preclude operative intervention. Type B dissections are most often treated with medical therapy, but stent grafting or surgery may be recommended depending on the clinical circumstance [2].

References

1. Chen K, Varon J, Wenker OC, *et al.* Acute thoracic aortic dissection: the basics. *J Emerg Med.* 1997;15:859–6.
2. Verhoye JP, Miller DC, Sze D, *et al.* Complicated acute type B aortic dissection: midterm results of emergency endovascular stent-grafting. *J Thorac Cardiovasc Surg* 2008;136:424–30.

4 Aortic Intramural Hematoma

Jing Ping Sun[1], Xing Sheng Yang[1] & Joel M. Felner[2]

[1] Emory University School of Medicine; Emory University Hospital Midtown, Atlanta, GA, USA
[2] Grady Memorial Hospital; Emory University School of Medicine, Atlanta, GA, USA

History

A 50-year-old man complains of an episode of nausea, vomiting, and diaphoresis.

Physical Examination

Blood pressure was 60/30 mmHg; heart rate was 50/minute and was regular. He was given 2 L of intravenous fluids en route to the hospital and all the symptoms were resolved completely.

Laboratory

The magnetic resonance imaging raised the suspicion of an intramural hematoma in the ascending aorta (AAO). This finding was also seen on computed tomography.

Transesophageal echocardiography (TEE) suggested an intramural hematoma in the posterior aspect of AAO (Figure 4.1 and Videoclip 4.1). No dissection flap or intraluminal compromise was noted.

Discussion

Aortic intramural hematoma (IMH) is an acute, potentially lethal disorder that is similar to, but pathologically distinct from, acute aortic dissection. In this condition, there is hemorrhage into the aortic media in the absence of an intimal tear. An autopsy study [1] noted that 13% of patients with a diagnosis of aortic dissection had IMH. These hematomas, like thoracic aortic dissections, involve the ascending aorta, such as in our case, aortic arch or both termed type A or the descending aorta named type B [2]. Although intimal disruption is not present, the prognosis is similar to that of classic aortic dissection; therefore, early diagnosis is critical.

Underlying medial degeneration is the possible pathogenesis of IMH. Other risk factors for IMH, such as bicuspid aortic valve, Marfan

Practical Handbook of Echocardiography 1st edition. Edited by Jing Ping Sun, Joel Felner and John Merlino. © 2010 Blackwell Publishing Ltd.

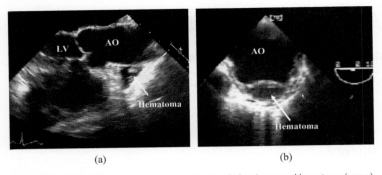

Figure 4.1. Transesophageal echocardiography revealed an intramural hematoma (arrow) intraposterior aspect of ascending aorta in the long-axis view (a), and short-axis view (b). No dissection flap or intraluminal compromise was noted. AO, aorta; LV, left ventricle.

syndrome, and collagen vascular disease, have been uncommon in cases of IMH.

Echocardiography has become an important modality for the diagnosis of aortic IMH. TEE is remarkably accurate in the detection of intimal flaps [3].

Several studies have demonstrated that bleeding in the media layer of the aorta evolves dynamically in the short term, and may be reabsorbed or progress to classical dissection or aortic rupture [4]. The optimal therapy for IMH is uncertain. In patients with descending IMH without rupture or compromised organ perfusion, medical therapy will be appropriate.

References

1. Wilson SK, Hutchins GM. Aortic dissecting aneurysms: causative factors in 204 subjects. *Arch Pathol Lab Med* 1982;106:175–9.
2. Nienaber CA, von Kodolitsch Y, Petersen B, *et al.* Intramural hemorrhage of the thoracic aorta. Diagnostic and therapeutic implications. *Circulation* 1995;92:1465–72.
3. Kang D, Song J, Song M, *et al.* Clinical and echocardiographic outcomes of aortic intramural hemorrhage compared with acute aortic dissection. *Am J Cardiol* 1998;8:202–6.
4. Shimizu H, Yoshino H, Udagawa H, *et al.* Prognosis of aortic intramural hemorrhage compared with classic aortic dissection. *Am J Cardiol* 2000;85:792–5.

5 Giant-Cell Arteritis

Jing Ping Sun[1], Xing Sheng Yang[1] & Joel M. Felner[2]

[1] Emory University School of Medicine; Emory University Hospital Midtown, Atlanta, GA, USA
[2] Grady Memorial Hospital; Emory University School of Medicine, Atlanta, GA, USA

History

A 30-year-old female has a history of myocardial infarction (MI) and severe aortic regurgitation (AR) due to ostial left main coronary stenosis secondary to giant cell vasculitis.

Physical Examination

Cardiovascular exam was significant for tachycardia, with 3/6 systolic and diastolic murmurs.

Laboratory

The hemoglobin and hematocrit were 7.7 and 22.9 respectively. A blood test revealed an increased erythrocyte sedimentation rate.

Echocardiography

Transthoracic echocardiography (TTE): Homogeneous thickening aortic wall was seen on ascending aorta long-axis view, which caused aortic valve stenosis (AS). The diameter of the aortic root was 0.45 cm during systole with high-velocity color flow. The peak velocity through the stenosis area was 317 cm/sec and the gradient was 41.2 mmHg (Figure 5.1). Transesophageal echocardiography (TEE): Homogeneous thickening aortic wall was seen on short-axis view of aortic root (Figure 5.1a, Videoclip 5.1a), which caused AS and AR (Videoclip 5.1b). There is a floating mass appearing vegetation in the ascending aortic long-axis view, also can be seen in the aortic short-axis view (Videoclip 5.2).

Discussion

Giant cell arteritis (GCA) is the most common systemic vasculitis. Ischemic manifestations are well known. In cases of thoracic aortic

Practical Handbook of Echocardiography 1st edition. Edited by Jing Ping Sun, Joel Felner and John Merlino. © 2010 Blackwell Publishing Ltd.

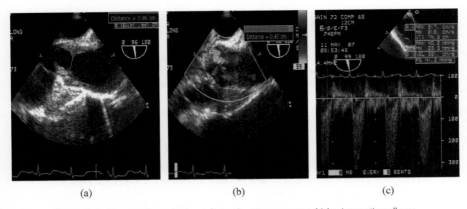

(a)   (b)   (c)

Figure 5.1. Transesophageal echocardiography: Homogeneous thickening aortic wall was seen on ascending aorta long-axis view, which caused the aortic stenosis (a), the diameter of aortic root is 0.45 cm during systole with high-velocity color flow (b). The peak velocity through the stenosis area was 317 cm/sec and the gradient was 41.2 mmHg (c).

aneurysms with unknown etiology, GCA is a possible cause. GCA is an inflammation of the lining of the arteries. Most often, it affects the arteries in the head, especially those in temples. For this reason, GCA is sometimes called temporal arteritis or cranial arteritis. GCA frequently causes headaches, jaw pain, and blurred or double vision, less often blindness and chest pain in rare cases [1].

Complications of GCA may occur years after the initial diagnosis; the aorta should be monitored with annual chest X-ray, ultrasound, computed tomography (CT) scan or MRI (magnetic resonance imaging) [1, 2]. A blood clot may form in an affected artery, obstructing blood flow completely and causing stroke. In our case, giant cell arteritis involved the aorta and left main coronary artery, which complicated with myocardial infarction, AS, and AR.

To confirm a diagnosis of GCA is by taking biopsy from the temporal artery.

Treatment for GCA consists of high doses of a corticosteroid drug such as prednisone, usually relieves symptoms and may prevent loss of vision. The patients should start feeling better within days of starting treatment, but it may need to continue taking medication for 1–2 years or longer [1].

References

1. Mayo Clinic foundation. Giant cell artiritis. *Mayo Clin Proc* 2008;83:1–3.
2. Hunder GG, Bloch DA, Michel BA, *et al.* The American College of Rheumatology 1990 criteria for the classification of giant cell arteritis. *Arthritis Rheum* 1990;33:1122.

Part 2
Aortic Valvular Diseases

6 Quantification of Aortic Regurgitation Using Echocardiography

Jing Ping Sun & Alicia N. Rangosch
Emory University School of Medicine; Emory University Hospital Midtown, Atlanta, GA, USA

Aortic regurgitation (AR) is characterized by diastolic reverse of blood from the aorta into left ventricle (LV) due to malcoaptation of the aortic cusps. Its clinical presentation is variable and depends on a complex interplay of a number of factors, including acuity of onset, aortic and LV compliance, hemodynamic conditions, and severity of the lesion.

In acute aortic regurgitation (AR), immediate surgical intervention is necessary because the acute volume overload results in life-threatening hypotension and pulmonary edema [1].

Patients with chronic AR may be asymptomatic for many years or even for their entire life.

The difficult issue is when to operate on asymptomatic patients to prevent irreversible LV dysfunction. Outcomes are better in patients with an LV ejection function (LVEF) >55% or an end-systolic LV diameter <55 mm (or <25 mm/m^2) [2,3]. Careful, serial echocardiographic follow-up is necessary to identify patients for surgery before their LV values reach these thresholds.

The causes of AR have different implications with regard to treatment, such as bicuspid aortic valve, degenerative aortic valve disease, aortic root dilation, endocarditis, and dissection of the ascending aorta.

Echocardiography is the most important diagnostic test for evaluation of AR. The anatomy of the aortic leaflets and the aortic root, the presence and severity of AR, and characterization of LV size and function can be assessed and detected by 2D and color Doppler echocardiography.

The American Society of Echocardiography guidelines for quantification of valvular regurgitation emphasize the need to integrate all of this information to properly evaluate patients with AR.

It is important to quantify the severity of AR for surgical decision making. Doppler color flow mapping is widely used to identify the presence of AR and estimate its severity. In general, color flow jets consist of three distinct components. The proximal area of flow acceleration into the orifice is the flow convergence zone, the narrowest and highest velocity region of the jet at or just downstream from the orifice named the vena contracta, and the jet itself occurs distal to the orifice in the LV cavity [Figure 6.1, Videoclip 6.1].

Practical Handbook of Echocardiography 1st edition. Edited by Jing Ping Sun, Joel Felner and John Merlino. © 2010 Blackwell Publishing Ltd.

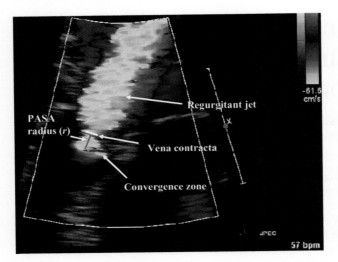

Figure 6.1. The proximal area of flow acceleration into the orifice is the flow convergence zone, the narrowest and highest velocity region of the jet at or just downstream from the orifice named the vena contracta, and the jet itself occurs distal to the orifice in the left ventricular cavity.

There are several methods to estimate the severity of AR using echocardiography.

1. The jet width/left ventricular outflow tract (LVOT) width ratio method: Perry *et al.* [4] compared the ratio of AR jet width to LVOT width in a parasternal long-axis view to angiography. A jet width/LVOT width <25% is specific for mild AR, whereas a jet width/LVOT width ratio >65% is specific for severe AR (Figure 6.2). This works best when the regurgitant orifice is relatively round in shape. When it is elliptical, as in bicuspid aortic valves, this ratio can lead to underestimation of AR severity [5]. The short-axis view is helpful in identifying such cases.

2. *Vena contracta*: It is defined as the narrowest central flow region of a jet. In AR, it can be measured in a parasternal long-axis or short-axis view in a color Doppler mode (Figure 6.3). Tribouilloy *et al.* [6] demonstrated that a vena contracta width of ≥6 mm correlates well with severe AR, having a sensitivity of 95% and a specificity of 90%, conversely, a vena contracta width <3 mm is specific for mild AR in a study with 79 patients. The advantages of this method are simple, quantitative, and good at identifying mild to severe AR. The limitation is not useful in multiple jets.

3. *Proximal isovelocity surface area method*: Compared with MR, it is less common to identify a clear proximal flow convergence in AR. However, when it is present, the Nyquist velocity should be shifted toward the direction of the jet to produce a clearly visible, round proximal isovelocity surface area (PISA) region that is as large as possible. The surface area of the PISA region is $2\pi r^2$, where r is the radius from the

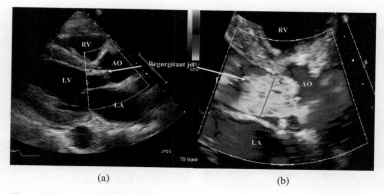

(a)   (b)

Figure 6.2. Perry *et al.* defined that a jet width/left ventricular outflow tract width <25% is specific for mild aortic regurgitation, whereas a jet width/left ventricular outflow tract width ratio >65% is specific for severe aortic regurgitation. The examples are color flow images from parasternal long-axis views in patients with mild (aortic regurgitation width/left ventricular outflow tract width = 21%) (a), and severe (aortic regurgitation width/left ventricular outflow tract width = 84%) aortic regurgitation (b). AO, aorta; LA, left atrium; LV, left ventricle; RV, right ventricle.

alias line to the orifice. Peak regurgitant flow (RF) is obtained by multiplying this value by the aliasing velocity (Va), which convert to formula is RF = $(2\pi r^2 \times Va)$. The effective regurgitant orifice area (EROA) is the peak regurgitant flow divided by the peak velocity (PVar) obtained by continuous wave Doppler, The formula is ROA = $(2\pi r^2 \times Va)/PVar$. How to calculate this in a case is shown in Figure 6.4. The EROA < 0.1 cm^2 is defined as mild, ≥0.3 cm^2 as severe regurgitation.

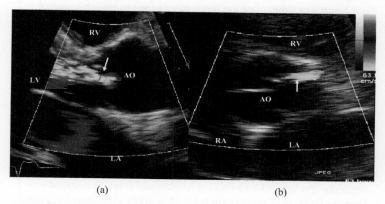

(a)   (b)

Figure 6.3. The vena contracta is seen as the narrowest part of the jet (arrow) as it emerges from the regurgitant orifice; it is better to measure from parastenal long-axis views (a) or apical views. The short-axis view (b) is difficult to orient precisely in the plane of the vena contracta but is useful in determining whether the jet is central and round or markedly elliptical (in which the long-axis vena contracta may underestimate aortic regurgitation severity). AO, aorta; LA, left atrium; LV, left ventricle; RA, right atrium; RV, right ventricle.

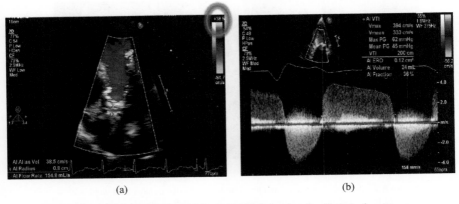

(a)   (b)

Figure 6.4. Color Doppler recording from apical five-chamber view illustrates how to calculate the effective regurgitant orifice using round proximal isovelocity surface area method (a). The r value was 0.8, Va 38.5, and peak velocity of aortic regurgitation was 394 cm/sec in this case (b). The effective regurgitant orifice area (EROA) can be calculated according to the formula EROA = $(2\pi \times r^2 \times Va)/PVAR$, and regurgitant volume (RV) = EROA × VTI$_{AR}$. EROA = $(3.1416 \times 2 \times 0.64 \times 38.5)/394 = 0.39$ cm^2. The EROA < 0.1 cm^2 is defined as mild, ≥ 0.3 cm^2 as aortic regurgitation.

The PISA method has been shown to work in AR but is less accurate in eccentric jets or aortic root dilation [7].

4. *Quantitative Doppler flow measurements*: AR volume and fraction can be calculated by comparing flow at the aortic level with that at the mitral valve level [8]. The stroke volume is generally obtained by area of left ventricular out tract (LVOT area = πr^2) times the velocity time integral (VTI) of pulsed Doppler LVOT flow. The mitral stroke volume is measured in similar fashion but is more prone to error because of difficulty in accurately measuring the mitral annulus. Measuring mitral stroke volume, the pulsed Doppler sample volume should be placed at the level of mitral annulus.

The AR volume is the difference between stroke volume of the mitral valve and forward stroke volume of the aortic valve. The cut points for AR severity measured by regurgitant volume are <30 mL/beat defined as mild, ≥60 mL/beat as severe. The regurgitant fraction is regurgitant volume divided by stroke volume of aortic valve, these cut points for AR severity are <30% defined as mild, ≥50% as severe. According to the formula-regurgitant volume (RV) = EROA × VTI$_{AR}$, effective regurgitant orifice area (EROA) can be calculated by dividing the regurgitant volume (RV) by VTI$_{AR}$ jet obtained from continuous wave Doppler (VTI$_{AR}$). The equation is EROA = RV/VTI$_{AR}$, these cut points are <0.1 cm^2 for mild, and ≥0.3 cm^2 for severe.

Another method is by assuming that an excess of the aortic volume flow (AF) compared with the pulmonary volume flow (PF) is due to aortic regurgitant flow. The aortic regurgitant fraction (RF) was calculated as follows: RF(%) = (AF − PF)/AF × 100.

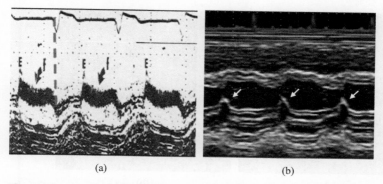

(a)   (b)

Figure 6.5. M-mode recording indicates the mitralanterior valvular flutter (arrows) (a), and early mitral valve closure (arrows) indicates increased left ventricular filling pressures and is often present in severe aortic regurgitation (b).

The mean Doppler-determined aortic regurgitant fraction was 2.4% for normal subjects, 28.0% for the patients with 1+, 32.6% for the patients with 2+, 53.3% for the patients with 3+, and 62.4% for the patients with 4+ [9]

5. *Supportive findings*: A number of echocardiographic findings provide supporting evidence for AR severity.
   - M-mode echocardiography, early mitral valve closure indicates increased LV filling pressures and is often present in severe AR (Figure 6.5), unless masked by tachycardia.
   - The continuous wave Doppler spectral signal of the AR jet provides clues to the severity of the leak. With severe AR, diastolic pressure will decrease rapidly in the aorta, thus leading to a shorter pressure half-time or more rapid deceleration slope (Figure 6.6). As a general rule, an AR pressure half-time <200 msec indicates severe AR,

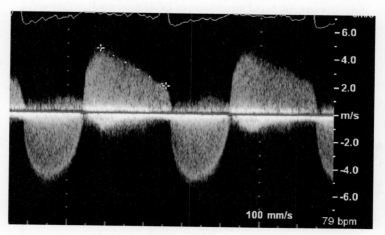

Figure 6.6. Continues wave Doppler recording shows the pressure half time: mild aortic regurgitation > 500 msec, severe aortic regurgitation < 200 msec.

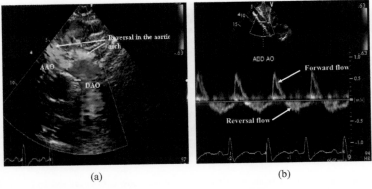

(a)   (b)

Figure 6.7. Aortic arch image with Color Doppler illustrates a holodiastolic flow reversal usually indicating at least moderate aortic regurgitation (a). Diastolic flow reversal in the abdominal aorta recorded with pulsed-wave Doppler (b). AAO, ascending aorta; ABDA, abdomen aorta; DAO, descending aorta.

whereas a pressure half-time >500 msec suggests mild AR. The pitfalls are that the eccentric jets, sinus tachycardia, atrial fibrillation and conditions that alter LV compliance and aortic diastolic pressures are the factors that will influence the accuracy of this method.
- Another important supportive sign of severe AR is diastolic flow reversal in the descending aorta. Although brief early diastolic flow reversal is often seen in normal subjects, holodiastolic flow reversal usually indicates at least moderate AR. Diastolic flow reversal in the descending aorta is best measured with pulsed-wave Doppler (Figure 6.7)
6. *Left ventricle size and geometry*: LV dimensions, volumes, and ejection fraction (EF) are important determinants of the need for surgery in chronic severe AR. Serial progression of LV dilation predicts the need for surgery [3]. It is important to establish a link between severity of AR and LV dysfunction, because LV chamber dilation and systolic dysfunction can occur from other causes. Repeated echocardiography to assess progression of LV dilation and severity of AR is recommended every 2–3 years in stable asymptomatic patients with normal LV size and function. In asymptomatic patients with LV dilation, more frequent echocardiography (every 6–12 months) is indicated [3].

References

1. Cohn LH, Birjiniuk V. Therapy of acute aortic regurgitation. *Cardiol Clin* 1991;9:339–52.
2. Bonow RO, Carabello B, de Leon AC Jr, *et al.* ACC/AHA guidelines for the management of patients with valvular heart disease: a report of the American College of Cardiology/American Heart Association Task Force on Practice Guidelines. *J Am Coll Cardiol* 1998;32:1486–588.
3. Borer JS, Bonow RO. Contemporary approach to aortic and mitral regurgitation. *Circulation* 2003;108:2432–8.

4. Perry GJ, Helmcke F, Nanda NC, Byard C, Soto B. Evaluation of aortic insufficiency by Doppler color flow mapping. *J Am Coll Cardiol* 1987;9:952–9.
5. Taylor AL, Eichhorn EJ, Brickner ME, *et al.* Aortic valve morphology: an important in vitro determinant of proximal regurgitant jet width by Doppler color flow mapping. *J Am Coll Cardiol* 1990;16:405–12.
6. Tribouilloy CM, Enriquez-Sarano M, Bailey KR, Seward JB, Tajik AJ. Assessment of severity of aortic regurgitation using the width of the vena contracta: a clinical color Doppler imaging study. Circulation 2000;102:558–64.
7. Meyer T, Sareli P, Pocock WA, *et al.* Echocardiographic and hemodynamic correlates of diastolic closure of mitral valve and diastolic opening of aortic valve in severe aortic regurgitation. *Am J Cardiol* 1987;59:1144–8.
8. Grayburn PA, Handshoe R, Smith MD, Harrison MR, DeMaria AN. Quantitative assessment of the hemodynamic consequences of aortic regurgitation by means of continuous wave Doppler recordings. *J Am Coll Cardiol* 1987;10:135–41.
9. Kitabatake A, Ito H, Inoue M, *et al.* A new approach to noninvasive evaluation of aortic regurgitant fraction by two-dimensional Doppler echocardiography. *Circulation* 1985;72:523–9.

7 Aortic Stenosis

Jing Ping Sun[1] & Joel M. Felner[2]

[1] Emory University School of Medicine; Emory University Hospital Midtown, Atlanta, GA, USA
[2] Grady Memorial Hospital; Emory University School of Medicine, Atlanta, GA, USA

The causes of aortic stenosis include (1) congenitally bicuspid valve; (2) rheumatic heart disease; and (3) degenerative changes in the valve. Examples of different causes of aortic stenosis are shown in Figure 7.1 and Videoclip 7.1.

Echocardiography

Two and three-dimensional echocardiography provides the image (transesophageal echocardiography or TEE is better than transthoracic echocardiography or TTE) to measure the aortic valve area and to evaluate the extent of leaflet calcification.

Other findings on the echocardiogram that may be helpful in the assessment of severity include patterns of leaflet motion; when leaflets move together in a "dome-like" pattern, the possibility of significant obstruction (or bicuspid valve) is increased. In significant stenosis cases, poststenotic dilatation is usually present. The varying degrees of concentric left ventricle hypertrophy (LVH) may present. The examples of cases with severe aortic stenosis are shown in Figure 7.2 and Videoclip 7.2.

Doppler echocardiography quantification of transaortic systolic pressure gradient and valve area is required for the definitive diagnosis [1]. It is essential to position continuous wave Doppler probe in a number of sites including the apex, suprasternal notch, and right parasternal intercostal spaces. This enables to record the highest velocity.

When the highest velocity is recorded, the simplified Bernoulli equation can be applied to obtain the peak instantaneous gradient: Peak pressure gradient (mmHg) = $4 \times$ peak velocity^2 (Figure 7.3).

According to the AHA/ACC Guidelines (2008), the standards of grading the degree of stenosis using definitions of aortic jet velocity, mean pressure gradient, and valve area are as follows [2]:

Indicator	Mild	Moderate	Severe
Jet velocity (m/sec)	Less than 3.0	3.0–4.0	Greater than 4.0
Mean gradient (mmHg)	Less than 25	25–40	Greater than 40
Valve area (cm^2)	Less than 3.0	1–1.5	Less than 1.0

Practical Handbook of Echocardiography 1st edition. Edited by Jing Ping Sun, Joel Felner and John Merlino. © 2010 Blackwell Publishing Ltd.

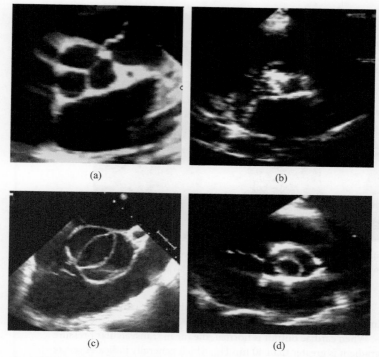

Figure 7.1. Normal trileaflet aortic valve (a), aortic valvular stenosis caused by thickened and calcified trileaflet valve (b), bicuspid aortic valve (c), and unicuspid aortic valve (d).

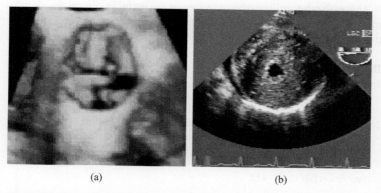

Figure 7.2. Three-dimensional image shows thickened and stenotic aortic valve (a). Transesophageal echocardiographic image shows a hypertrophied left ventricle due to severe aortic stenosis (b).

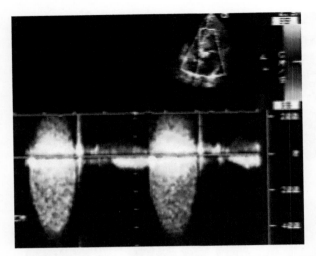

Figure 7.3. Doppler recording shows the high-velocity trans through aortic valve (4.5 m/sec, with a calculated peak gradient of 81 mmHg), which indicates a severe aortic stenosis.

Normalization for body surface area should be considered in those individuals at the extremes of body size.

When cardiac output is normal, the mean transvalvular pressure gradient is greater than 40 mmHg, which generally indicates severe stenosis. However, when patients with severe aortic stenosis (AS), left ventricle (LV) systolic dysfunction, and a low cardiac output often present with only modest transvalvular pressure gradients (less than 30 mmHg).

Some patients with severe AS remain asymptomatic, whereas others with only moderate stenosis develop symptoms.

Although echocardiographic assessments are useful in clinical decision making, it should be combined with symptoms to determine the optimum timing of valve replacement surgery.

References

1. Godley, RW, Green, D, Dillon, JC, *et al.* Reliability of two-dimensional echocardiography in assessing the severity of valvular aortic stenosis. *Chest* 1981;79:657.
2. Bonow RO, Carabello BA, Chatterjee K, *et al.* American College of Cardiology/American Heart Association Task Force on Practice Guidelines. 2008 focused update incorporated into the ACC/AHA 2006 guidelines for the management of patients with valvular heart disease. *J Am Coll Cardiol* 2008 September;52(13):e1–142.

Part 3
Mitral Valvular Diseases

8 Isolated Cleft Mitral Valve in Adult

Xing Sheng Yang, Jing Ping Sun & John D. Merlino

Emory University School of Medicine; Emory University Hospital Midtown, Atlanta, GA, USA

History

A 50-year-old male is presented with tiredness and atypical chest pain.

Physical examination was unremarkable except for a regular grade 3/6 systolic murmur heard on the mitral valve area.

Laboratory

Transthoracic echocardiography (TTE) demonstrated a grade 3 to 4+ mitral regurgitation (MR) due to two separate mitral valve orifices (Figure 8.1, Videoclip 8.1), dilated left atrium (LA) and mild left ventricle (LV) enlargement with good contractility. The cleft of the mitral anterior leaflet is well seen in parasternal long-axis (PLA) view (Figure 8.1). Mitral valve had dysplastic leaflets (Figure 8.2, Videoclip 8.2). The valve had a triangular opening, with the anterior leaflet divided into two by a cleft in parasternal short-axis (PSA) view (Figure 8.3, Videoclip 8.3).

Discussion

Mitral valve clefts not associated with a septal defect of the endocardial cushion type septal defect, also called isolated cleft mitral valve (ICMV), is a rare, well-recognized cause of congenital mitral insufficiency [1]. In a report of 20 patients with ICMV, the median age at presentation was 3.8 years (15 days to 12.7 years) [2]. Our patient may be the oldest one among reported cases. Most commonly, the cleft involves the mitral anterior leaflet. An association with other cardiac anomalies such as secundum-type atrial septal defect, transposition of the great arteries, ventricular septal defect (VSD), tricuspid atresia, patent ductus arteriosus (PDA), coarctation of the aorta, double outlet RV and anomalous pulmonary venous connection have been previously described [3]. At younger ages, clefts cause mild mitral insufficiency. Perier *et al.* [4] studied

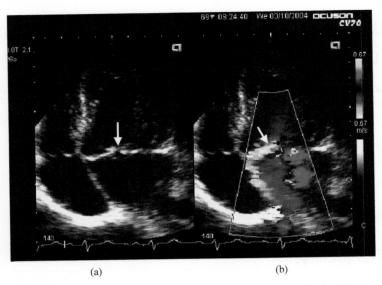

(a)   (b)

Figure 8.1. (a) A4-ch view illustrates a cleft (arrow) of the mitral anterior leaflet. (b) Color Doppler recording shows a mitral regurgitation jet (arrow) passing through the cleft into the left atrium.

older patients and detected more severe degrees of MR, suggesting some worsening with age, as happened in our 50-year-old patient. In the present case, the cleft was not identified in childhood, and the MR worsened in subsequent years, with need for cardiac surgery. Because the MR in ICMV appears to be progressive, early surgical treatment is indicated even when MR is mild [2]. The treatment consists of direct suturing of the cleft.

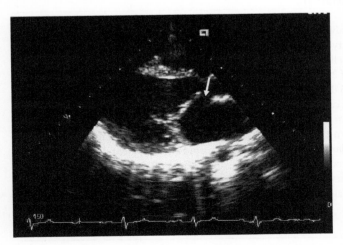

Figure 8.2. The cleft (arrow) of the mitral anterior leaflet is well seen in parasternal long-axis view.

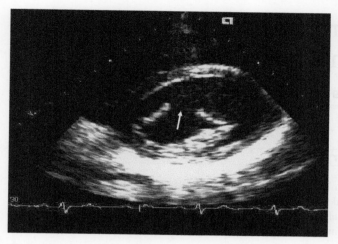

Figure 8.3. Parasternal long axis view shows a cleft (arrow) of the anterior mitral leaflet.

References

1. Di Segni E, Kaplinsky E, Klein H. Color Doppler echocardiography of isolated cleft mitral valve. Roles of the cleft and the accessory chordae. *Chest* 1992;101:12–15.
2. Tamura M, Menahem S, Brizard C. Clinical features and management of isolated cleft mitral valve in childhood. *J Am Coll Cardiol* 2000;35:764–70.
3. McDonald RW, Ott GY, Pantely GA. Cleft in the anterior and posterior leaflet of the mitral valve: a rare anomaly. *J Am Soc Echocardiogr* 1994;7:422–4.
4. Perier P, Clausnizer B. Isolated cleft mitral valve: valve reconstruction techniques. *Ann Thorac Surg* 1995;59:56–9.

9 Mitral Valve Prolapse in Case with Atrial Septal Defect

Jing Ping Sun & Xing Sheng Yang
Emory University School of Medicine; Emory University Hospital Midtown, Atlanta, GA, USA

History

A 40-year-old male with a several-year-history of Huntington's disease presented with a syncopal episode 2 days ago.

Physical examination: Blood pressure was 120/78 mmHg with grade 3/6 systolic murmur at the apex.

Laboratory

Two-dimensional echocardiography revealed left ventricle hypertrophy (LVH); left ventricle (LV) cavity size was moderately increased with normal systolic function. Both mitral leaflets extended superior to a line connecting the annular hinge points in the parasternal long-axis (PLA) view with moderate mitral regurgitation (MR) (Figure 9.1a, Videoclip 9.1). Three-dimensional echocardiography showed mitral valve prolapse (MVP) clearly (Figure 9.2). A small secundum atrial septal defect was detected from the subcostal and A4-ch views with left to right shunt (Videoclip 9.2).

For comparison, we put another case with mitral posterior leaflet prolapse in Figure 9.3 and Videoclip 9.2.

Discussion

Isolated MVP is observed in 2.5–5% of the general population. The incidence is higher in women than in men [1]. Classic MVP is due to myxomatous degeneration.

The rate of observing MVP in patients with atrial septal defect (ASD) varies between 35 and 95% in various studies [2]. Right ventricle (RV) volume loading, dilatation and paradoxical septal movement have been observed in patients with ASD. As a result, MVP is functional in patients with ASD [3].

Practical Handbook of Echocardiography 1st edition. Edited by Jing Ping Sun, Joel Felner and John Merlino. © 2010 Blackwell Publishing Ltd.

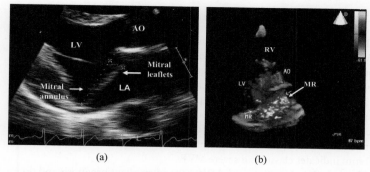

Figure 9.1. Both mitral leaflets extend superior to a line connecting the annular hinge points (dash line) in the parasternal long-axis view (a). Three-dimensional color Doppler recording shows the width of mitral regurgitation in the parasternal long-axis view (b). AO, aorta; LA, left atrium; LV, left ventricle; MR, mitral regurgitation; RV, right ventricle.

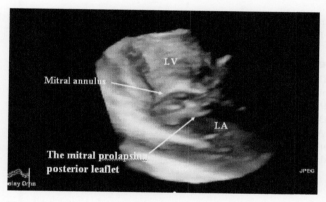

Figure 9.2. Three-dimensional echocardiography shows mitral valve prolapse. LA, left atrium; LV, left ventricle.

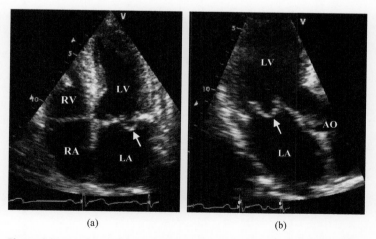

Figure 9.3. Apical 4-chamber view shows the mitral posterior leaflet extends superior to a line connecting the annular hinge points (arrow) (a). The apical long-axis view shows the mitral posterior leaflet prolapse (b). AO, aorta; LA, left atrium; LV, left ventricle; RA, right atrium; RV, right ventricle.

Echocardiography is the most useful noninvasive test for diagnosing MVP. On 2D echocardiography, systolic displacement of one or both mitral leaflets in the PLA view, particularly when they coaptate on the atrial side of the annular plane, indicates MVP.

Three-dimensional echocardiography is particularly valuable as it allows visualization of the mitral leaflets relative to the mitral annulus. This allows measurement of the leaflet thickness and its displacement relative to the annulus. Thickening of the mitral leaflets >5 mm and leaflet displacement >2 mm indicates classic and severe MVP.

The majority of patients with MVP have an excellent prognosis and do not need treatment. For these individuals, routine examination including echocardiogram every 3–5 years is recommended. Patients with a normal appearance of the valves and without regurgitation do not need prophylaxis.

Symptomatic patients, those with evidence of LV dilatation and diminished function need urgent attention.

References

1. Savage DD, Garrison RJ, Devereux RB, *et al.* MVP in the general population. 1. Epidemiologic features: the Framingham study. *Am Heart J* 1983;106:571–6.
2. Jeresaty RM. Mitral valve prolapse-click syndrome in atrial septal defect. *Chest* 1975;67:132–3.
3. Weyman AE, Wann S, Feigenbaum H; Dillon JC. Mechanism of abnormal septal motion in patients with right ventricular volume overload: a cross-sectional echocardiographic study. *Circulation* 1976;54:179–86.

10 Mitral Valve Aneurysm

Jing Ping Sun[1] & Joel M. Felner [2]

[1] Emory University School of Medicine; Emory University Hospital Midtown, Atlanta, GA, USA
[2] Grady Memorial Hospital; Emory University School of Medicine, Atlanta, GA, USA

History

A 40-year-old male presented with acute bacterial endocarditis and was treated with intravenous antibiotics for 8 weeks.

Cardiovascular Examination

He was afebrile with a normal heart rate of 90. Blood pressure (BP) was 138/66 mmHg.

Auscultation: a grade 3/6 holodiastolic murmur, at the right second inter space, and a grade 2/6 short, systolic murmur were audible at the apex.

Laboratory

Transthoracic echocardiography (TTE) revealed severe aortic regurgitation (AR), a trileaflet aortic valve with a small vegetation on the noncoronary cusp, moderate mitral regurgitation (MR), and mild tricuspid regurgitation (TR). Left ventricle (LV) was dilated with an ejection fraction (EF) of 55%. A suspicious aneurysm was present on the mitral valve (Figure 10.1a,b; Videoclip 10.1a,b,c).

Transesophageal echocardiography (TEE) confirmed the above findings and revealed an aneurysm on the anterior mitral leaflet (Figure 10.1c,d; Videoclip 10.1c,d). MR was present and flow entered but did not traverse the aneurysm (Figure 10.2; Videoclip 10.2a,b,c).

Hospital Course

The patient underwent operation of aortic valve replacement, and the mitral valve was inspected through a left atriotomy. A 2- to 3-cm saccular aneurysm was identified on the anterior leaflet of mitral valve corresponding to A2 and A3. There were no vegetations or atrial thrombi visible. The aneurysm was excised and the leaflet repaired by oversewing its base.

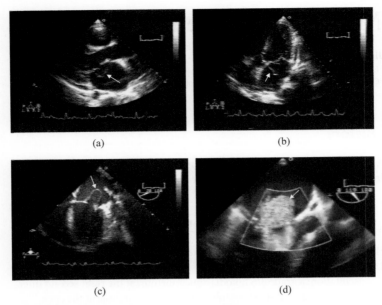

Figure 10.1. Transthoracic echocardiography: (a) parasternal long-axis view shows mitral aneurysm (arrow). (b) Apical 5-chamber view shows the aneurysm from anterior leaflet (arrow). TEE:(c) At a 32° angle view, the image shows the mitral valve aneurysm (arrow). (d) At a 119° angle view, color Doppler shows the regurgitate flow enveloped by the aneurysm (arrow).

Postoperative TEE revealed normal coaptation of the mitral valve leaflets with no MR or AR. He was discharged on the fourth postoperative day. After 6 months, he remains asymptomatic with good mitral valve function as demonstrated on TEE.

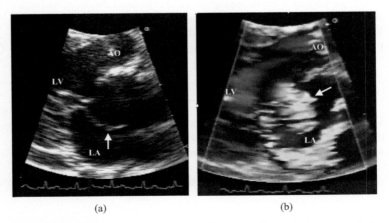

Figure 10.2. Transthoracic echocardiography: (a) parasternal long-axis view shows mitral aneurysm (arrow). (b) Same view with color Doppler shows the mitral valve regurgitant flow enveloped by the aneurysm (arrow). AO, aorta; LA, left atrium; LV, left ventricle.

Pathology

Pathologic analysis of the aneurysm revealed myxomatous change with fresh fibrin dissecting the midportion of the valve.

Discussion

Aneurysms of the mitral valve are rare complications of aortic valve endocarditis. The cause of the aneurysm is most likely a combination of occult infection of the mitral valve leaflets and leaflet weakening due to the high velocity regurgitant jet associated with AR. Subclinical infection may occur by direct extension of the infectious process from the aortic valve or by seeding of the mitral leaflets from AR [1]. Because mitral valve aneurysms rarely occur in the absence of endocarditis or in patients with pure AR, an infectious etiology is at least partly responsible for leaflet degeneration.

The histologic findings of the resected specimen, and the discovery of the mitral valve aneurysm in association with the infected aortic valve indicate that the aneurysm in our case was caused by aortic valve endocarditis.

TTE may occasionally identify subtle valvular abnormalities, but TEE yields a more definitive identification. Color Doppler distinguishes the aneurysm from these other abnormalities by demonstrating direct communication between the aneurysm and LV [2].

Echocardiographic follow-up of these lesions has demonstrated progressive expansion and subsequent rupture with development of acute MR. Therefore, in patients with mitral valve aneurysms, repair or replacement of the valve should be performed during aortic valve replacement.

References

1. Reid CL, Chandraratna PAN, Harrison E, *et al.* Mitral valve aneurysm: clinical features, echocardiographic-pathologic correlations. *J Am Coll Cardiol* 1983;2:460–64.
2. Vilacosta I, San Roman JA, Sarria C, *et al.* Clinical, anatomic and echocardiographic characteristics of aneurysms of the mitral valve. *Am J Cardiol* 1999;84:110–13.

11 Mitral Valve Stenosis

Jing Ping Sun[1] & Joel M. Felner[2]

[1] Emory University School of Medicine; Emory University Hospital Midtown, Atlanta, GA, USA
[2] Grady Memorial Hospital; Emory University School of Medicine, Atlanta, GA, USA

A standard echocardiographic examination of the mitral valve consists of an M-mode tracing, multiple two-dimensional (2D) views, and Doppler flow evaluation [1]. If clinically indicated (e.g., technically difficult transthoracic imaging or evaluation of prosthetic paravalvular leak), a transesophageal echocardiography (TEE) may be performed.

The *M-mode* diagnosis of mitral valve stenosis (MS) is based on an increase in echo production from the thickened, deformed, often calcified leaflets; a decrease in the opening amplitude of the valve; anterior motion of the posterior leaflet; and a decrease in the diastolic or EF slope (Figure 11.1a).

Two-dimensional echocardiography: MS alters the 2D appearance of the valve because it partially fuses the normally independent leaflets; an increase in echo production from the thickened, deformed mitral leaflets; a reduction in mitral orifice area; and creates persistent gradient between the left ventricle (LV) and left atrium (LA). This gradient keeps the stenotic diastolic orifice opened to its maximum and causes the entire valve to dome or bulge into the ventricle throughout diastole. In the parasternal short axis plane, the opening of the valve can be imaged just above the tips of the papillary muscles. From this orientation, its maximum diastolic opening area (Figure 11.2a and Videoclip 11.1a) can be measured by direct planimetry of the 2D image. This method is a reliable means of judging the severity of obstruction [2]. Typically, a valve orifice area of <1 cm^2 is considered severe, <1.5 cm^2 as moderate, and >1.5 cm^2 as mild mitral valve stenosis [3].

Severe dilated LA with spontaneous echo contrast may be present (Figure 11.2b and Videoclip 11.1b).

Three-dimensional echocardiography: transesophageal echocardiography (TTE) and TEE were performed expeditiously and with adequate quality (92 and 93% respectively). Accuracy between the methods (3D TEE and TTE, 2D TEE and TTE) and surgical findings were 96, 90, 87, 77%, respectively [4]. Am example is shown in Figure 11.2c,d.

Doppler echocardiography provides a constellation of measurements to estimate which the severity of MS. These variables include the gradient across the valve, the inferred area by the pressure half-time, the continuity equation or the proximal flow convergence, and the pulmonary pressure at rest and during exercise from the tricuspid regurgitant jet velocity [5].

Practical Handbook of Echocardiography 1st edition. Edited by Jing Ping Sun,
Joel Felner and John Merlino. © 2010 Blackwell Publishing Ltd.

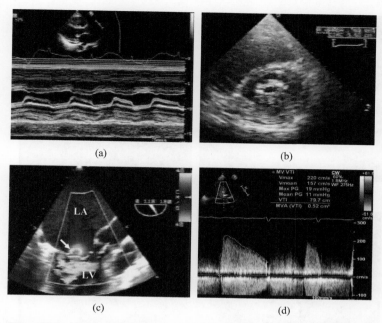

(a)   (b)

(c)   (d)

Figure 11.1. (a) M-mode recording illustrates thickened, deformed, and calcified mitral leaflets in the opening amplitude of the valve and anterior motion of the posterior leaflet. (b) Parasternal short-axis view illustrates diffuse thickening of the leaflet tips and marked reduction in mitral valve orifice area. (c) Color flow mapping (transesophageal echocardiography) displays the acceleration field proximal to a stenotic mitral valve (arrow). (d) Continuous wave Doppler recording shows the peak and mean velocity are higher, indicating mitral valve stenosis. LA, left atrium; LV, left ventricle.

In MS, the velocity of mitral inflow increases at rest from a normal value of less than 1 m/sec to greater than 1.5 m/sec. The algorithm to convert Doppler velocity into pressure gradient is the modified Bernoulli equation. Peak gradient, in mmHg $= 4 \times$ peak velocity^2.

The mean transmitral gradient can be measured by tracing the velocity time integral of mitral inflow E and A waves (by continuous wave). The 2008 ACC/AHA guidelines on valvular heart disease defined severe MS as a mean transmitral gradient >10 mmHg (Figure 11.2d). Pulmonary artery systolic pressure >50 mmHg, and a mitral valve area <1 cm^2 [3].

The pressure half-time is the time required for the gradient between the LA and LV to fall to one-half of its initial value. In order to convert Doppler velocity into a pressure gradient, the initial flow velocity is divided by 1.41 (square root of 2), because velocity bears a second order relationship to pressure. Empirically, a pressure half-time of 220 msec is equivalent to a mitral valve area (MVA) of 1 cm^2, therefore,

$$MVA = \frac{220}{\text{pressure half} - \text{time}}$$

Calculating the MVA using the pressure half-time may be an inaccurate approach whenever abrupt changes in the transmitral gradient occur for

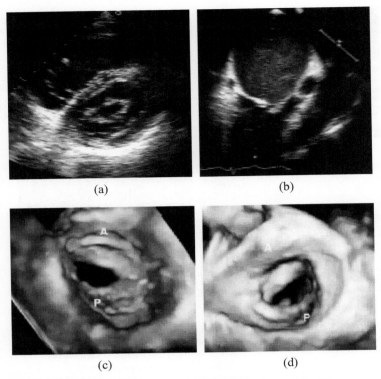

(a) (b)

(c) (d)

Figure 11.2. (a) parasternal short-axis view shows the stenotic mitral valve. (b) transesophageal echocardiography shows the stenotic mitral valve and dilated left atrium with smoke. (c) Three-dimensional images show a thickened and stenotic mitral valve from the left ventricular side, and (d) from the left atrial side.

reasons other than inflow obstruction. An example of such a change is additional ventricular filling from aortic regurgitation.

Among the methods for estimating MS severity, direct planimetry of the orifice is probably the most accurate when performed correctly. However, in a clinical setting, it is the universal practice to achieve cross validation by applying all of the echocardiographic methods.

Indirect methods to identify the severity of MS include estimating the extent of leaflet calcification (Videoclip 11.1a), the degree of LV underloading (i.e., volume decrease), the presence of RV and RA dilatation (Videoclip 11.1b), and the degree of tricuspid regurgitation and pulmonary hypertension, as determined by Doppler of tricuspid regurgitant jet.

Treatment: If untreated, MS often progresses to significant symptoms (dyspnea and fatigue), serious complications (pulmonary edema, systemic arterial embolism, pulmonary hypertension, and death). Medical therapy can relieve symptoms but does not affect the obstruction to flow. Patients with severe symptomatic MS have demonstrated a significant reduction in mortality with surgery compared to medical therapy [6]. Surgical approaches include closed commissurotomy, open commissurotomy, mitral valve repair, and mitral valve replacement. When correction of MS is indicated, the question remains which surgical option, if any, is most appropriate for a given patient, especially in light of the success achieved with percutaneous mitral balloon valvotomy (PMBV). Images of PMBV are shown in Videoclip 11.2b.

In clinical trials comparing open commissurotomy to PMBV in patients who are candidates for valvotomy, the outcome was as good (Videoclip 11.2c) or better after PMBV [7]. Other advantages of PMBV are shorter hospital stay, avoidance of the morbidity of thoracotomy, and a better outcome if repeat intervention is required [8]. Open commissurotomy with valve repair remains an appropriate choice in patients who are not candidates for PMBV due to valve deformity or calcification, left atrial thrombus, or significant MR.

The 2006 ACC/AHA guidelines reached the following conclusions: Surgery is indicated in patients with New York Heart Association (NYHA) class III or IV symptoms and, on Doppler echocardiography, a mean mitral valve gradient greater than 10 mmHg. Surgery is a weaker recommendation in two settings: patients with mild (NYHA class II) symptoms and, on Doppler echocardiography, a mean mitral valve gradient greater than 10 mmHg; in asymptomatic patients with a pulmonary artery systolic pressure ≥50 mmHg and, on Doppler echocardiography, a mean mitral valve gradient ≥10 mmHg [3].

The efficacy of surgery was not well established in asymptomatic patients with new onset atrial fibrillation or multiple systemic emboli despite adequate antithrombotic therapy.

References

1. Marcus RH, Sareli, P, Pocock WA, Barlow JB. The spectrum of severe rheumatic valve disease in a developing country. *Ann Intern Med* 1994;120:177.
2. Nichol PM, Gilbert BW, Kisslo JA. Two-dimensional echocardiographic assessment of MS. *Circulation* 1977;55:120.
3. Bonow RO, Carabello BA, Chatterjee K, *et al.* American College of Cardiology/American Heart Association Task Force on Practice Guidelines. 2008 focused update incorporated into the ACC/AHA 2006 guidelines for the management of patients with valvular heart disease. *J Am Coll Cardiol* September 2008;52(13):e1–142.
4. Pepi M, Tamborini G, Maltagliati A, *et al.* Head-to-head comparison of two- and three-dimensional transthoracic and transesophageal echocardiography in the localization of mitral valve prolapse. *J Am Coll Cardiol* 2006;48:2524.
5. Tischler MD, Niggel J. Exercise echocardiography in combined mild mitral valve stenosis and regurgitation. *Echocardiography* 1993;10:453.
6. Dahl, JC, Winchell, P, Borden, CW. MS. A long term postoperative follow-up. *Arch Intern Med* 1967;119:92.
7. Reyes VP, Raju BS, Wynne J, *et al.* Percutaneous balloon valvuloplasty compared with open surgical commissurotomy for MS. *N Engl J Med* 1994;331:961.
8. Reyes VP, Raju BS, Wynne J, *et al.* Percutaneous balloon valvuloplasty compared with open surgical commissurotomy for MS. *N Engl J Med* 1994;331:961.

12 Quantification of Mitral Regurgitation

Jing Ping Sun & Alicia N. Rangosch

Emory University School of Medicine; Emory University Hospital Midtown, Atlanta, GA, USA

The mitral apparatus includes leaflets, chordae tendineae, annulus, papillary muscles, and their supporting left ventricular walls. The malfunction of any part of the mitral apparatus can cause mitral regurgitation (MR). The anatomy picture of the mitral valve is shown in Figure 12.1. The etiology of MR divided as primary: include mitral valve prolapse, infective endocarditis, trauma, rheumatic heart disease, and congenital heart disease; and secondary: include ischemic heart disease, left ventricular systolic dysfunction, hypertrophic cardiomyopathy, degenerative valve, and mitral annulus disease.

Mitral valve prolapse is the most common cause of primary MR in developed countries and is degenerative or myxomatous mitral valve disease.

Trauma can cause ruptured chordae and acute MR. Rheumatic heart disease is uncommon in developed countries but continues to constitute a significant burden in the rest of the world. Rheumatic mitral valve disease is more frequent in women than men and disease detection is higher by echocardiography compared to clinical examination.

A variety of congenital anomalies of the mitral valve can cause MR, for example, a cleft anterior or posterior mitral leaflet. Mitral annular calcification is a common finding in older adults that is often associated with mild to moderate MR.

Pathophysiology

Acute phase:
- The left atrium (LA) and left ventricle (LV) do not have the opportunity to gradually enlarge and compensate for the volume overload
- LA pressure rises and the patient develops congestive heart failure with diminished cardiac output and pulmonary venous congestion. Most patients with severe acute mitral regurgitation require emergency surgical intervention.

Subacute compensated phase:
- Eccentric left ventricle hypertrophy and increased-end diastole volume

---

Practical Handbook of Echocardiography 1st edition. Edited by Jing Ping Sun, Joel Felner and John Merlino. © 2010 Blackwell Publishing Ltd.

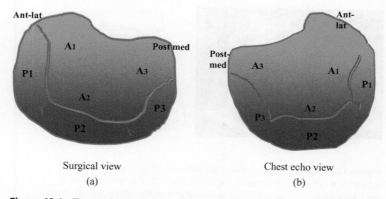

Surgical view
(a)

Chest echo view
(b)

Figure 12.1. The mitral valve anatomy: The post mitral leaflet is widest around the annulus and has three scallops: P1, P2, and P3. P1 is adjacent to the anterolateral commissure and is closest to the aorta (anterior). The opposing sections of the anterior leaflet are designated A1, A2, and A3 (surgical view (a), chest echo view (b)). Ant-lat, anterolateral.

- Normal ejection fraction (EF) allows the ejection of a sufficiently large stroke volume that makes the forward stroke volume return toward normal despite the fraction being regurgitated
- LA enlarges to accommodate the regurgitant volume and can maintain a lowered filling pressure.

Chronic phase:
- LV and LA enlargement
- End systole volume increases
- End diastole pressure increases
- Pulmonary congestion

Mechanisms of MR

- Failure to coapt (perforation, annulus dilatation, cleft)
- Excessive leaflet motion (prolapse, flail leaflet, chordal rupture)
- Restriction leaflet motion (chordal shortening and fusion, leaflet stiffness)

Determination of severity: Over 20 variables for judging the severity of MR have been described [1]. Through the employment of this approach severe lesions are readily recognized, but distinguishing among the intermediate grades of MR (mild to moderate, moderate to severe mitral regurgitation) can be more difficult.

Echocardiography is essential for establishing the etiology and hemodynamic consequences of MR. Other important echocardiographic features are LA and LV size, systolic function, and pulmonary artery pressures. LA size is usually increased. LV size and systolic function are normal early in the disease course but progressive ventricular dilation and a decline in EF occur with chronic severe regurgitation. ACC/AHA 2006

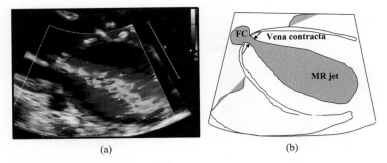

(a)   (b)

Figure 12.2. (a) Parasternal long axis view with color Doppler shows the mitral regurgitation (MR). (b) The corresponding picture illustrates the components of the regurgitant jet: flow convergence (FC), vena contracta, and jet area in the left atrium.

guidelines for the management of patients with valvular heart disease, consensus statement on management of valvular heart disease [2], recommended using multiple parameters when determining the severity of mitral regurgitation. These parameters include structural, color Doppler, and quantitative Doppler parameters.

Structural parameters: Structural abnormalities associated with MR supplement the quantitation of regurgitation and include LA and LV size, and appearance of the mitral apparatus.

- Mild MR is usually associated with normal or near-normal LA and LV size, and intact mitral apparatus.
- Moderate MR is frequently associated with some degree of LA enlargement, normal or mildly dilated LV, and varying degrees of mitral apparatus abnormalities.
- Severe chronic MR is usually associated with moderate to severe LA enlargement, some degree of LV dilatation, and often associated with flail mitral leaflet, ruptured papillary muscle, or malcoaptation of the mitral leaflets.

Color flow Doppler: The features of severe mitral regurgitation seen by color flow Doppler imaging arise from the high energy transfer of a volume of blood into LA, producing the characteristic "jet" in LA (Figure 12.2). Color flow Doppler is usually considered a quantitative or semiquantitative parameter.

In current practice, there are three-color Doppler methods to estimate the severity of MR.

Jet area: To trace LA and jet area, and calculate the percentage of jet area/LA area. (Figure 12.3, 12.4)

- Mild MR: small central jet <4 cm^2 or <20% of LA area
- Severe MR: jet area > 40% of LA or an eccentric jet of any size, whirling in LA

Vena contracta of MR: (1) to measure the width of the neck or narrowest portion of the jet (Figure 12.5) and adjust to high resolution,

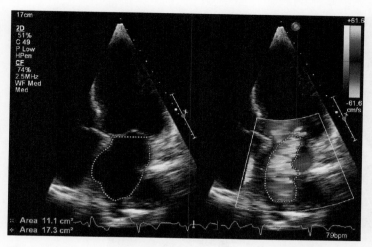

Figure 12.3. Apical 4-chamber view without and with color Doppler illustrates the measurement of the left atrium and jet area.

high-frequency rate and zoom images; (2) to use multiple planes and measure the largest obtainable proximal jet size.

- Mild mitral regurgitation: vena contracta <0.3 cm
- Severe mitral regurgitation: vena contracta ≥0.7 cm

The regurgitant orifice in MR may not be circular, and is often elongated along the mitral coaptation line (Figure 12.6). The MR is often dynamic

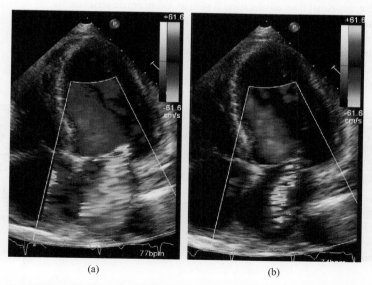

(a)   (b)

Figure 12.4. Apical 4-chamber views show an example with severe mitral regurgitation (jet area > 40% of left atrium or an eccentric jet of any size, whirling in left atrium) (a), and a case with mild mitral regurgitation (small central jet < 4 cm² or <20% of left atrial area) (b) estimated by jet and left atrial area.

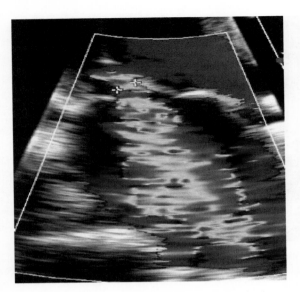

Figure 12.5. An apical 3-chamber view with color Doppler shows vena contracta width. Mild mitral regurgitation: vena contracta width <0.3 cm. Severe mitral regurgitation: vena contracta width ≥0.7 cm

and therefore the vena contracta may change with hemodynamics or during systole

Proximal isovelocity surface area or PISA: On the ventricular side of the valve, proximal flow acceleration is seen as a concentric series of hemispheric rings of alternating colors, each ring denoting an isovelocity of aliasing [3]. To obtain apical 3- or 4- chamber view, optimize flow convergence, zoom and adjust the aliasing velocity (color baseline down) such that a well-defined hemisphere is shown. To measure the diameter of the ring from the first aliasing shell to base of the hemisphere.

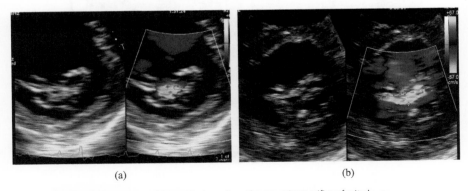

(a)   (b)

Figure 12.6. Parasternal long-axis views show the regurgitant orifice of mitral regurgitation may not be circular (a) and is often elongated (b) along the mitral coaptation line. The mitral regurgitation is often dynamic and therefore the vena contracta may change with hemodynamics or during systole.

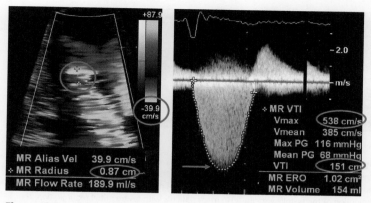

Figure 12.7. The figures illustrate the calculation of mitral regurgitant (MR) orifice area (MroA) and volume (Rvol). The equations are MroA = (6.28 r^2Va)/Vmax reg; Rvol = MroA × VTI$_{MR}$. In this case: r = 0.87, Va = 39.9, Vmax reg = 538, and VTI$_{MR}$ = 151 cm; the calculation of MroA was 1.02 cm² and the mitral regurgitation volume was 154 mL. Mild mitral regurgitation = MroA < 0.20 cm². Severe mitral regurgitation = MroA ≥ 0.4 cm².

The Figure 12.7 illustrates the calculation of mitral regurgitant (MR) orifice area (MroA) and volume (Rvol). The equations are:

$$\text{MroA} = \frac{(6.28\ r^2\,Va)}{\text{Vmax reg}};\ \text{Rvol} = \text{MroA} \times \text{VTI}_{MR}$$

Mild MR = MroA of < 0.20 cm²; Rvol of ≤ 30 mL/beat

Moderate MR = MroA of 0.2 − 0.39 cm²; Rvol of 30 − 59 mL/beat

Severe MR = MroA of ≥ 0.4 cm²; Rvol of ≤ 60 mL/beat

Pulsed and continuous wave Doppler of mitral inflow: Spectral Doppler recognition of severe MR also has many diagnostic features. In severe decompensated mitral regurgitation, the tricuspid regurgitation peak velocity will be increased as the result of pulmonary hypertension.

In the case with solo mitral regurgitation (without aortic valve regurgitation), the flow quantization (PW Doppler) also can be used to calculate the mitral regurgitant orifice and volume. The equations are:

Stroke volume (SV) = Cross section area (CSA) × Flow velocity integral (VTI).

Mitral regurgitant volume (MRV) = SVmv − SVav

$$\text{Mitral regurgitant fraction (MRF)} = \frac{\text{MRV}}{\text{SVmv}}$$

$$\text{Mitral Regurgitant Orifice Area (MroA)} = \frac{\text{Regurgitant Volume}}{\text{VTImr}}.$$

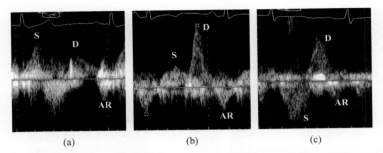

(a)   (b)   (c)

Figure 12.8. Pulse Doppler recording of pulmonary vein: (a) Normal pulmonary venous flow is characterized by a velocity during ventricular systole (S) that is higher than during ventricular diastole (D). (b) With increasing severity of mitral regurgitation, there is a diminution of the systolic velocity. (c) In many patients with severe mitral regurgitation, the flow in the pulmonary veins becomes reversed in systole. AR, aortic regurgitation.

In the equation: mv = mitral valve, av = aortic valve and mr = mitral regurgitation, calculation of flow and stroke volume through the mitral valve with pulsed Doppler is performed by placing the sample volume at the mitral annulus level.

Doppler of pulmonary veins: Doppler interrogation of the pulmonary veins has produced insights into hemodynamics. In mitral regurgitation, this evaluation is a standard part of the examination and usually includes pulse Doppler of the left and right upper pulmonary veins from the apical four-chamber view. Normal pulmonary venous flow is ante grade during both ventricular systole (S) and diastole (D) (ventricular systolic component dominates), with slight retrograde flow during atrial systole (AR). In hemodynamically severe mitral regurgitation, the flow in one or more pulmonary veins (depending upon the direction of the jet) will show systolic flow reversal (Figure 12.8).

References

1. Schiller NB, Foster E, Redberg RF. Transesophageal echocardiography in the evaluation of mitral regurgitation. The twenty-four signs of severe mitral regurgitation. *Cardiol Clin* 1993;11:399.
2. Bonow RO, Carabello BA, Chatterjee K, *et al.* ACC/AHA 2006 guidelines for the management of patients with valvular heart disease. A report of the American College of Cardiology/American Heart Association Task Force on Practice Guidelines (writing committee to revise the 1998 guidelines for the management of patients with valvular heart disease). *J Am Coll Cardiol* 2006;48:e1.
3. Utsunomiya T, Doshi R, Patel D, *et al.* Regurgitant volume estimation in patients with mitral regurgitation: initial studies using color Doppler "proximal isovelocity surface area" method. *Echocardiography* 1992;9:63.

Part 4
Prosthetic Valves

13 Mitral Valve Repair with the Use of an Annuloplasty Ring: The Importance of Echocardiography

Joel M. Felner[1] & Jing Ping Sun[2]

[1] Grady Memorial Hospital; Emory University School of Medicine, Atlanta, GA, USA
[2] Emory University School of Medicine; Emory University Hospital Midtown, Atlanta, GA, USA

Mitral valve repair, referred to as valvuloplasty, is preferred for the surgical treatment of mitral regurgitation (MR) [1]. It almost always involves placing a ring at the mitral orifice that is either rigid or flexible. Ring sizes most commonly used are 30 mm and 32 mm. The causes of MR referred for valvuloplasty are as follows: degenerative disease (75%), postischemic disease (10%), rheumatic valvular disease (5%), and infectious endocarditis (5%).

The echocardiography images obtained from a case had degenerative MR repaired with the use of the annuloplasty ring with normal function shown in Figure 13.1 and Videoclip 13.1. Transesophageal echocardiography (TEE) recordings from a case, who had a vegetation was seen on the mitral valve repaired with an annuloplasty ring, and MR demonstrated by color Doppler (Figure 13.2 and Videoclip 13.2).

Preoperative echocardiography can identify structural features of the mitral valve that aid in the selection of the appropriate surgical procedure. Transthoracic echocardiography (TTE) and TEE have identified the following features that favor repair: (1) limited calcification of the leaflets or annulus; (2) prolapse of less than one-third of the leaflet; (3) pure annular dilatation; (4) valvular perforations; and (5) incomplete papillary muscle rupture. TEE is essential in the operating room to better define the anatomy, ensure an adequate repair, and confirm the absence of complications after repair [2].

By performing TTE in the long axis, the maximum anteroposterior diameter of the mitral valve ring in diastole (Dd), the smallest diameter in systole (Ds), and left ventricle end-diastolic dimension (LVED) can be determined. The percentage of shortening of the mitral valve ring in systole (delta D%) and ratio Dd/LVED can also be calculated. Mitral annular motion has been examined by means of the extent of the mitral annulus systolic excursion, as measured in four longitudinal LV segments (anterior, inferior, septal, and lateral). Mean and peak transmitral flow velocities can also be evaluated by continuous-wave Doppler [3].

Practical Handbook of Echocardiography 1st edition. Edited by Jing Ping Sun, Joel Felner and John Merlino. © 2010 Blackwell Publishing Ltd.

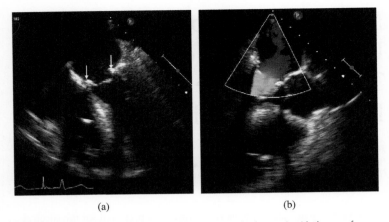

(a)   (b)

Figure 13.1. Transesophageal echocardiography: mitral valve repair with the use of an annuloplasty ring (arrows) (a), with normal function by color Doppler (b).

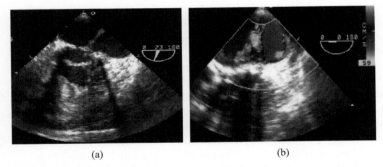

(a)   (b)

Figure 13.2. Transesophageal echocardiography: a vegetation was seen on the mitral valve repaired with an annuloplasty ring (a), and mitral regurgitation demonstrated by color Doppler (b).

References

1. Enriquez-Sarano M, Freeman WK, Tribouilloy CM, *et al.* Functional anatomy of mitral regurgitation: accuracy and outcome implications of transesophageal echocardiography. *J Am Coll Cardiol* 1999;4:1129–36.
2. Hellemans IM, Pieper EG, Ravelli AC, *et al.* Prediction of surgical strategy in mitral valve regurgitation based on echocardiography. *Am J Cardiol* 1997;7:334–8.
3. Bonow RO, Carabello BA, Chatterjee K, *et al.* ACC/AHA 2006 guidelines for the management of patients with valvular heart disease. *J Am Coll Cardiol* 2006;48:e1.

14 Biological Prostheses Valves

Jing Ping Sun[1] & Joel M. Felner[2]

[1] Emory University School of Medicine; Emory University Hospital Midtown, Atlanta, GA, USA
[2] Grady Memorial Hospital; Emory University School of Medicine, Atlanta, GA, USA

History

A 30-year-old male presented with acute heart failure secondary to streptococcus *milleri* endocarditis two months ago. At his initial presentation, both the mitral and aortic valves were involved with severe mitral regurgitation (MR) and aortic regurgitation (AR). He underwent emergency mitral and aortic valve replacements with bioprosthetic valves. He was treated with intravenous antibiotics for 1 month and discharged. Two weeks later after discharge, he developed paroxysmal palpitations associated with shortness of breath without fever or chills.

Physical Examination

There was a holosystolic murmur at the cardiac apex with no extra cardiac sounds.

Laboratory

The first transthoracic echocardiography (TTE) performed before this admission: The left ventricle (LV) was significantly dilated with normal systolic function. There were several vegetations on the aortic and mitral valves causing severe AR and MR (Figure 14.1, 14.2 and Videoclip 14.1).

The echocardiography was performed at the time of this admission: The aortic valve bioprosthesis was normal (Figure 14.3 and Videoclip 14.2). Severe periprosthetic posterior directed jet of MR (Figure 14.4 and Videoclip 14.3). This jet is related to mitral prosthetic valve dehiscence. No vegetations were seen. The LV cavity was markedly increased in size with reduced contractility. Transesophageal echocardiography (TEE) revealed: no evidence of endocarditis. Dehiscense of the mitral valve was seen on both 2D and 3D images (Figure 14.5 and Videoclip 14.4). The aortic bioprosthesis valve is functioning well; there was no evidence of aortic valve endocarditis.

Practical Handbook of Echocardiography 1st edition. Edited by Jing Ping Sun, Joel Felner and John Merlino. © 2010 Blackwell Publishing Ltd.

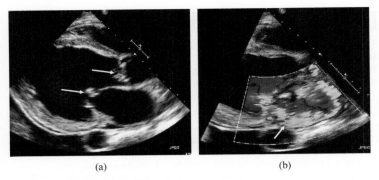

(a)   (b)

Figure 14.1. The vegetations on the aortic and mitral valves are seen in the PLA view (arrows) (a). The severe MR is demonstrated by color Doppler (arrow) (b).

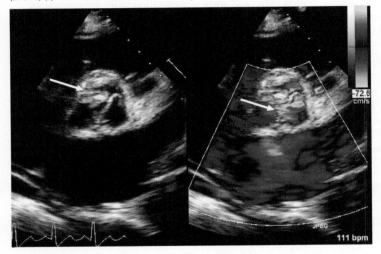

Figure 14.2. The vegetations on aortic valve are seen in the PSA view (arrow); the AR is demonstrated by color Doppler (arrow).

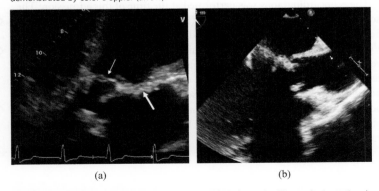

(a)   (b)

Figure 14.3. TEE revealed a normal Carpentier–Edwards porcine bioprosthetic aortic valve (thin arrow) and a thickened bioprosthetic mitral valve (thickened arrow) during diastole (a) and a normal Carpentier–Edwards porcine bioprosthetic aortic valve during systole (b).

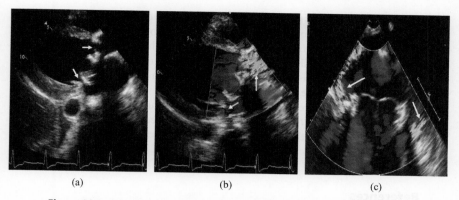

(a)   (b)   (c)

Figure 14.4. TTE: The dehiscence of biologic prosthetic valve (arrows) can be well seen in PLA view (a). The regurgitant flows (arrows) through two dehiscence areas are demonstrated by color Doppler (b). The regurgitant flows through two dehiscence areas are well seen by TEE color Doppler (c).

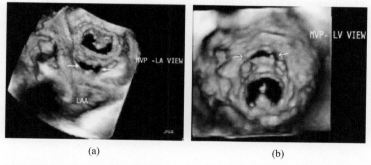

(a)   (b)

Figure 14.5. Three-dimensional short-axis views show the dehiscence areas (arrows) of biological mitral valve (left atrium (LA) view, (a); left ventricle (LV) view (b); LAA, left atrial appendage. MVP, mitral valve prolapse).

Discussion

TTE may help evaluate normal prosthetic valve function. Doppler echocardiography provides hemodynamic information with regard to prosthetic valve pressure gradient, is usually sufficient to exclude a stenotic valve. The normal gradient across a prosthetic valve depends upon the type, size, and position of the prostheses as well as the cardiac output [1].

The velocity of an apparently normal Carpentier–Edwards porcine mitral valve is 1.8 ± 0.2 m/sec, the maximal gradient is 12.5 ± 3.67 and mean gradient 6.5 ± 2.1 mmHg; aortic valve is 2.5 ± 0.5 m/sec, 23.2 ± 8.7 and 14.4 ± 5.7 mmHg. The velocity of a porcine prosthetic valve at the tricuspid position is 1.3 ± 0.3, the maximal gradient is 7 ± 2 and mean gradient 3 ± 2 mmHg [2].

Both TTE and TEE echocardiographic methods are complementary and should be used.

The complications of the biologic prosthetic valves are: (1) valve dysfunction resulting from a degenerative process – progressive leaflet thickening and calcification; as this process advances, the leaflet becomes more rigid and eventually develops fractures and tears or progressive stenosis; (2) endocarditis involving either the leaflets or the sewing ring; and (3) valve dehiscence.

In our patient the severe aortic and mitral valve dysfunction were caused by acute endocarditis. The biologic prosthetic valves were implanted at that time because endocarditis was acute. This resulted in sewing the valve into infective and very friable tissue that ultimately resulted in valve dehiscence 2 months later.

References

1. Faletra F, Constantin C, De Chiara F, *et al.* Incorrect echocardiographic diagnosis in patients with mechanical prosthetic valve dysfunction: correlation with surgical findings. *Am J Med* 2000;108:531.
2. Weyman AE. *Principle and Practice of Echocardiography*, 2nd edition. Philadelphia: Lea & Febiger, 1994, p. 1210.

15 Prosthetic Mechanical Valve

Jing Ping Sun[1] & Joel M. Felner[2]

[1]Emory University School of Medicine; Emory University Hospital Midtown, Atlanta, GA, USA
[2]Grady Memorial Hospital; Emory University School of Medicine, Atlanta, GA, USA

Transthoracic echocardiography (TTE) may help evaluate normal prosthetic valve function. Prominent acoustic shadowing that accompanies mechanical prostheses may limit transthoracic visualization of prosthetic leaflets, vegetations, abscesses, and thrombi [1]. The use of Doppler echocardiography that demonstrates normal transit prosthetic flow velocity and flow duration, is usually sufficient to exclude a stenotic valve. Exclusion of valvular regurgitation is more difficult, especially for mechanical prostheses in the mitral position. Doppler echocardiography provides hemodynamic information with regard to prosthetic valvular pressure gradients. The normal gradient across a prosthetic valve depends upon the type, size, and position of the prostheses as well as the cardiac output [1]. It is determined from the peak instantaneous transvalvular flow velocity using the modified Bernoulli equation ($\Delta P = 4v^2$).

A variety of mechanical valves are available including (1) a ball-cage valve; (2) a tilting-disk valve; and (3) a bileaflet valve.

The flow profiles through the mechanical valves are as follows:

- A ball-cage valve in the open position: The blood flows across the sewing ring and around the ball occluder on all sides. When the valve closes, a small amount of regurgitation is seen circumferentially around the ball.
- A tilting-disk valve: It is characterized by two orifices in the open position, one larger than the other with an asymmetric flow profile as blood accelerates along the tilted surface of the open disk.
- A bileaflet mechanical valve: It has complex fluid dynamics that affect the Doppler echocardiography's ability to evaluate these valves. In the open position, there are two large lateral valve orifices with a small narrow central orifice. The flow velocity profile shows three peaks corresponding to these three orifices (Figures 15.1 and 15.2; Videoclip 15.1).

Transthoracic echocardiography is usually sufficient for evaluation of an aortic prosthesis, but in the mitral position the atria are shadowed by a mechanical prosthesis. Transesophageal echocardiography (TEE), which images from a position posterior to the heart, allows the mitral valve to be seen. TTE demonstrates a ventricular side of the valve that lies in its near field, where as TEE does not. Both methods may have difficulty with the evaluation of the aortic prosthesis. Both echocardiographic methods should be used since they are complementary.

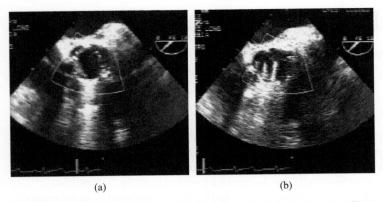

(a)   (b)

Figure 15.1. Normal St. Jude mechanical aortic valve prosthesis: Its two discs are well seen in diastole (a) and systole (b), respectively.

Prosthetic valvular regurgitation can arise from a variety of abnormalities, including dehisced sutures from a poorly seeded ring or from endocarditis. Severe hemolysis can occur after the mitral valve repair or replacement. To recognize a paravalvular leak, TEE should be performed using a Nyquist range of 35–50 cm/sec taken in several views (Videoclip 15.2). The most severe form of paravalvular regurgitation is seen when there is dehiscence of a substantial portion of the sewing ring. The sewing ring will rock with each cardiac cycle; mobile echo densities representing the suture material often may be seen. The TEE image obtained from a patient with an abnormal St. Jude mechanical mitral valve is shown in Figure 15.3 and Videoclip 15.3, which shows that one of the two discs is immobile.

Prosthetic valve stenosis is identified by a rise in transit prosthetic gradient across the prothetic valve from the baseline determination. Causes

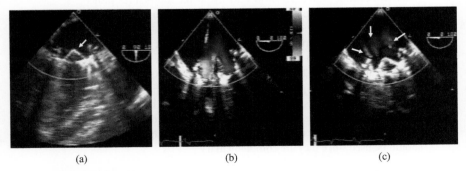

(a)   (b)   (c)

Figure 15.2. Normal St. Jude mechanical mitral valve prosthesis: Its two discs (arrow) are well seen (a). Color flow image of a normal St. Jude mechanical mitral valve in diastole shows acceleration of flow across the valve with two large lateral orifices and a small central orifice (b). Three normal "wash" jets (arrows) are well seen in systole (c).

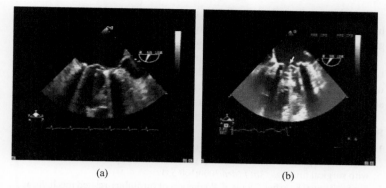

(a)   (b)

Figure 15.3. (a) Normal St. Jude mitral valve with its two discs is shown. (b) An abnormal St. Jude mechanical mitral valve shows that one of the two discs is immobile (arrow).

of obstruction include pannus in growth, thrombus, and vegetations. Finding spontaneous contrast in the left atrium without finding thrombus around the sewing ring in the setting of adequate anticoagulation should heighten suspicion of pannus formation. The most common etiology for prosthetic valve obstruction is thrombus formation. Pannus formation is far less common. Thrombus tends to be mobile, less echo dense and associated with spontaneous contrast. Pannus is highly echogenic and is usually firmly fixed to the valve apparatus [2].

Thromboemboli are prone to form on mechanical valves, and may result in systemic emboli or valve dysfunction. Transthoracic echocardiographic evaluation for thrombus is limited by shadowing and reverberations of the prosthetic valve. TEE is more sensitive, and should be performed when searching for thrombi in patients with mechanical valve. The TEE images of three patients with thrombi complications of bileaflet mechanical mitral or aortic valves are shown in Figure 15.4.

Endocarditis on a bioprosthetic valve may result in vegetation similar to that seen on a native valve. The infection on a mechanical valve, however, results in paravalvular leaks and a vegetation may not be present.

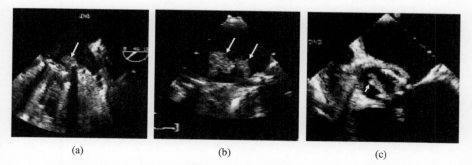

(a)   (b)   (c)

Figure 15.4. Transthoracic echocardiogram images of abnormal prosthetic valves: (a) a clot (arrow) is present on a St. Jude mechanical mitral valve; (b) two large clots (arrows) are seen on a mechanical mitral valve; and (c) a small clot is present on a St. Jude aortic valve.

Transthoracic Doppler echocardiography provides important hemodynamic information with regard to prosthetic valve pressure gradients and is extremely useful in long-term follow-up.

TEE has become an invaluable adjunct to transthoracic two-dimensional Doppler and color flow examination. It should be undertaken in all instances in which transthoracic information is not adequate, or if there is suspicion of an abnormality not detected by TTE.

References

1. Faletra F, Constantin C, De Chiara F, *et al.* Incorrect echocardiographic diagnosis in patients with mechanical prosthetic valve dysfunction: correlation with surgical findings. *Am J Med* 2000;108:531.
2. Lin SS, Tiong IY, Asher CR, *et al.* Prediction of thrombus-related mechanical prosthetic valve dysfunction using transesophageal echocardiography. *Am J Cardiol* 2000;86:1097.

16 Transcatheter Aortic Valve Replacement

Joel M. Felner[1], Jing Ping Sun[2] & Vasilus Babaliaros[2]

[1]Grady Memorial Hospital; Emory University School of Medicine, Atlanta, GA, USA
[2]Emory University School of Medicine; Emory University Hospital Midtown, Atlanta, GA, USA

The incidence of aortic stenosis rises as our life expectancy increases. In 2001, 0.8 million patients over the age of 65 had moderate to severe aortic stenosis. It is estimated that 1.8 million people will have aortic valve stenosis (AS) by the year 2050, approximately 2% of the population [1].

Nearly 200,000 people in the US need new aortic valves because of AS, yet over half of them do not receive this most effective treatment due to healthy condition [2].

Recently transcatheter methods have been used for aortic valve replacement to address this problem. Two techniques are under investigation: the retrograde transfemoral percutaneous approach performed by interventional cardiologists and the transapical minimally invasive approach performed by surgeons together with interventionalists. The Sapien Valve is presently being studied by both the transfemoral and transapical methods in the placement of aortic transcatheter valve (PARTNER) trial.

Optimal positioning of the prosthetic valve and the precise methods are critically important for avoiding embolization, paravalvular insufficiency, and coronary obstruction. Dependence on fluoroscopic visualization of the native valve is problematic owing to variability in the amount and location of calcification. Transesophageal echocardiography (TEE) is extremely useful in the positioning and determination of the aortic annulus size and root measurements. The procedure of percutaneous aortic valve replacement is shown in Videoclip 16.1. TEE images of the aortic valve (pre- and postprocedure) are shown in Videoclip 16.2. It often clarifies the relative positions of the prosthesis, annulus, and leaflets. The supra-annular aorta appears to play a less important role in valve securement. Ideal positioning appears to be dependent on prosthesis apposition with the annulus and outflow tract while extending just above the native leaflets. With accurate positioning, sizing, and deployment techniques, prosthesis embolization appears to be rare, as reflected in this initial apical access experience.

Since the initial demonstrations of the feasibility of percutaneous transarterial and transapical aortic valve replacement, this option has gained credibility as a viable alternative to open heart surgery in high-risk patients with symptomatic aortic stenosis.

Practical Handbook of Echocardiography 1st edition. Edited by Jing Ping Sun, Joel Felner and John Merlino. © 2010 Blackwell Publishing Ltd.

References

1. Nkomo VT, *et al.* Burden of valvular heart diseases: a population-based study. *Lancet* 2006;368:1005–11.
2. Iung B, *et al.* Decision-making in elderly patients with severe aortic stenosi: why are so many denied surgery? *Eur Heart J* 2005;26:2714–20.

Part 5
Coronary Artery Disease

17 Acute Myocardial Infarction Complicating Papillary Muscle Rupture

Xing Sheng Yang, Jing Ping Sun & John D. Merlino
Emory University School of Medicine; Emory University Hospital Midtown, Atlanta, GA, USA

History

A 76-year-old male presented to the emergency room with cardiogenic shock, acute renal failure, and acute myocardial infarction (AMI).

Laboratory

Cardiac catheterization revealed occlusion of the distal right coronary artery (RCA) and a 70% narrowing of the left main coronary artery (MCA). The patient was placed on an intra-aortic balloon pump and admitted to ICU. *Echocardiography*: The left ventricle (LV) and left atrium (LA) are dilated. The posterior wall reveals severe hypokinesis, and the posterior papillary muscle is completely transected (Figures 17.1a). Mitral valve prolapse is well seen in the A4-ch view during systole (Figure 17.1b, Videoclip 17.1). Severe mitral regurgitation (MR) is detected by color Doppler in A4-ch view (Videoclip 17.2).

Discussion

Papillary muscle rupture (PMR) following AMI leads to catastrophic outcomes [1]. It is important to recognize this complication early, because surgical repair is possible. In most cases, PMR causes <5% of ischemic MR; it usually occurs 2–7 days post AMI [2]. The incidence of PMR is 1% of all AMIs and accounts for 5% of the mortality following AMI. Thrombolytics have decreased its incidence; however, it tends to occur earlier [3]. PMR is more common in patients with inferior wall infarction, because the posteromedial papillary muscle is the single blood supply via the posterior descending coronary artery. The anterolateral papillary muscle has dual blood supply from both the left anterior descending and the left circumflex coronary arteries.

Practical Handbook of Echocardiography 1st edition. Edited by Jing Ping Sun, Joel Felner and John Merlino. © 2010 Blackwell Publishing Ltd.

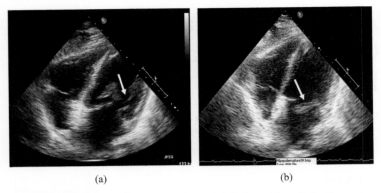

(a)   (b)

Figure 17.1. A4-ch view demonstrates: (a) the dilated left ventricle and left atrium and a complete transection of the posterior papillary muscle are well seen during diastole; (b) the posterior mitral valve prolapse is well seen during systole.

On auscultation, a new pansystolic murmur may be audible, but in severe cases the murmur may be soft or inaudible because of rapid equalization of LA and LV pressures.

Transthoracic views are usually adequate, but TEE may be required in some cases. Flail mitral leaflet or leaflets are often seen. The ruptured head or heads are seen to be attached to the leaflets by the mitral chordae. These can mimic vegetations, but the clinical presentation, the chordal attachment to the leaflets, and the usual attachment to both leaflets help to distinguish them from vegetations.

In patients with PMR following AMI, aggressive medical therapy with vasodilators, and emergent surgery with intra-aortic balloon pump as a bridge should be performed as soon as possible.

References

1. Hiroya M, Nobuhiko M, Hidefumi OBO. Papillary muscle rupture following acute myocardial infarction. *Jpn J Thorac Cardiovasc Surg* 2004;52:367–71.
2. Lehmann KG, Francis CK, Dodge HT. Mitral regurgitation in early myocardial infarction. Incidence, clinical detection, and prognostic implications. *Ann Intern Med* 1992;117:10–17.
3. Reeder GS. Identification and treatment of complications of myocardial infarction. *Mayo Clin Proc* 1995;70:880–84.

18 Ruptured Right Coronary Artery Aneurysm Resulting in Large Pseudoaneurysm

Jing Ping Sun, Erin Galbraith & Robert D. O'Donnell Jr.

Emory University School of Medicine; Emory University Hospital Midtown, Atlanta, GA, USA

History

A 57-year-old male on chronic dialysis was found incidentally on transthoracic echocardiography (TTE) to have a possible right atrial mass.

Physical Examination

Heart: Diastolic murmur at the upper sternal border and 2/6 mid-systolic murmur at the lower left sternal border radiating to the apex.

Laboratory

Echocardiography: There is a large cystic structure adjacent to the right atrium (RA) which is mildly compressed. It resembles a pericardial cyst. Several views suggest flow into cyst from RA, which suggests cyst cavity communicating with RA and RV (Figure 18.1 and Videoclip 18.1).

Magnetic resonance imaging (MRI) revealed a large rounded mass between the myocardium and pericardium lying in the lateral aspect of the right atrioventricular groove with flow into the mass (Videoclip 18.2). There was significant pericardial scarring and inferior left ventricle (LV) hypokinesis. Computed tomography (CT) angiogram revealed a mid right coronary artery (RCA) aneurysm that appeared to have ruptured distally causing a large pseudoaneurysm (Figure 18.2) and a fistula between the pseudoaneurysm and right ventricle (RV) through which the pseudoaneurysm was emptying its contents during diastole (Videoclip 18.3). The proximal and distal portions of the RCA were noted to be heavily calcified.

Treatment

Interventional cardiologist was consulted for the possibility of deploying a covered stent in the area of the aneurysm and pseudoaneurysm. It was unclear if a stent would be able to reach the area of interest or if it could be

Practical Handbook of Echocardiography 1st edition. Edited by Jing Ping Sun, Joel Felner and John Merlino. © 2010 Blackwell Publishing Ltd.

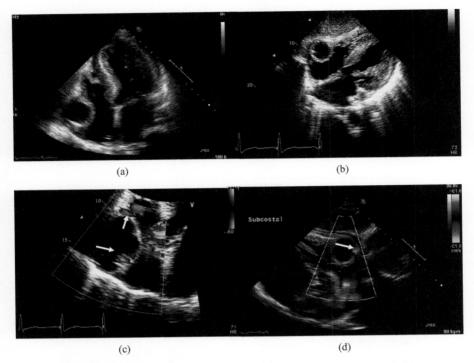

(a)   (b)

(c)   (d)

Figure 18.1. (a) There is a large cystic structure adjacent to the right atrium (RA) which is mildly compressed. (b) Subcostal 4-chamber shows a cyst. (c) A4-ch and (d) subcostal with color Doppler views suggest that there is communication flows between the cyst cavity and the right atrium.

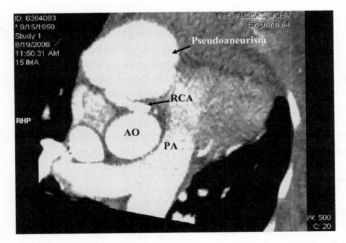

Figure 18.2. This large pseudoaneurysm is from the right coronary artery and is well demonstrated by CT image. AO, aorta; PA, pulmonary artery; RCA, right coronary artery.

deployed without further damaging the vessel and causing dissection. Given the potential risks of intervention, the patient opted to undergo repeat imaging in 1 month's time to assess for enlargement of the pseudoaneurysm. If there is evidence of expansion, she may undergo invasive coronary angiogram.

Discussion

Coronary aneurysms and pseudoaneurysms may occur spontaneously or as complications of various percutaneous coronary interventions. The incidence of spontaneous aneurysms is 1.5–2% on the basis of pre- and postmortem series [1], and 4.9% on the basis of the Coronary Artery Surgery Study registry [2].

Our patient has severe atherosclerotic coronary disease. She did have recent methicillin-resistant *Staphylococcus aureus* bacteremia and the possibility of her proximal RCA aneurysm having been mycotic, thus potentiating rupture with pseudoaneurysm development was hypothesized.

Spontaneous coronary artery pseudoaneurysm is a rare condition that has the potential risk of rupture or ischemia. Surgical repair and adequate coronary revascularization are reasonable for a coronary artery pseudoaneurysm [3].

The coronary artery pseudoaneurysm could not be clarified by TTE. In this case; MRI gave more information, and the complete diagnosis was best defined by CT.

References

1. Nishikawa H, Nakanishi S, Nishiyama S, *et al.* Primary coronary artery dissection observed at coronary angiography. *Am J Cardiol* 1988;61:645–8.
2. Swaye PS, Fisher LD, Litwin P, *et al.* Aneurysmal coronary artery disease. *Circulation* 1983;67:134–8.
3. Maehara A, Mintz GS, Castagna MT, *et al.* Intravascular ultrasound assessment of spontaneous coronary artery dissection. *Am J Cardiol* 2002;89:466–8.

19 Acute Myocardial Infarction Complicated by Ventricular Septal Perforation

Xing Sheng Yang, Jing Ping Sun & John D. Merlino
Emory University School of Medicine; Emory University Hospital Midtown, Atlanta, GA, USA

History

A 40-year-old male has a history of myocardial infarction (MI). He is noted to have a ventricular septal defect (VSD) demonstrated by catheterization and is admitted in preparation for possible surgery.

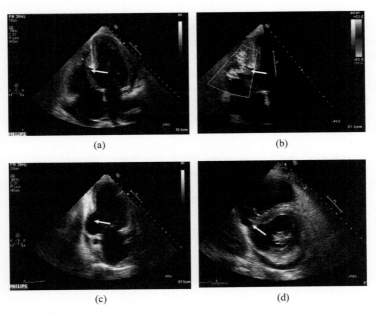

(a) (b)

(c) (d)

Figure 19.1. Apical 4-chamber view revealed a ventricular septal perforation (arrow, a); color Doppler shows a shunt through the septal perforation into right ventricle (RV) (arrow, b). An inferior wall aneurysm can be seen in apical 2-chamber view (arrow, c). A posterior septal perforation can be seen in the parasternal short-axis view (arrow, d).

Practical Handbook of Echocardiography 1st edition. Edited by Jing Ping Sun, Joel Felner and John Merlino. © 2010 Blackwell Publishing Ltd.

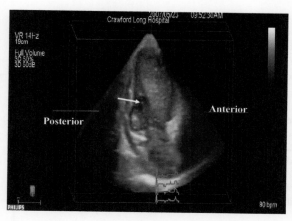

Figure 19.2. Three-dimensional transthoracic echocardiography: A circular clear area (arrow) in the inferior basal septum is noted in apical 2-chamber view that represents the septal perforation.

Physical Examination

Heart: A 2/6 holosystolic murmur was noted at the apex.

Echocardiography revealed that the left ventricle (LV) was moderately dilated. A posterior ventricular septal perforation with left to right shunt, and inferior wall aneurysm were noted in the apical 2-chamber and parasternal short-axis views (Figures 19.1, 19.2 and Videoclip 39.1). The shunt ratio was estimated at 2.3:1. The peak gradient across the defect was 82 mmHg. There was a small-to-moderate amount of pericardial effusion.

Surgical reduction of the aneurysm size and closure of the LV wall was carried out. The VSD was identified in the mid-septum posterior.

After the operation transthoracic echocardiography (TTE) demonstrated the LV size was normal and there was a small residual VSD.

Discussion

Ventricular septal perforation is a serious complication of acute myocardial infarction (AMI). Its incidence on autopsy has been estimated between 1 and 2% of all myocardial infarctions [1]. About 3% of transmural infarctions are complicated by septal perforation through a zone of necrotic myocardium [2], which occur mostly within the first week after AMI. Perforations are located in the anterior or apical portion of the ventricular septum in patients with anterior infarctions. Inferior infarction results in defects in the basal part of the septum [3]. Echocardiography is useful tool to evaluate LV aneurysms and allows early recognition of VSDs in the postinfarction patient with a new holosystolic murmur. A post infarct VSD can be recognized as an abrupt interruption in the septum with akinesis of the surrounding myocardium. If identification of the rupture site is difficult with 2D imaging, color Doppler can establish the diagnosis. A high-velocity left-to-right systolic jet is seen with continuous-wave Doppler, and systolic turbulence may be recorded on right ventricle (RV) side of the septum with color flow imaging. Transesophageal echocardiography may be useful if TTE is suboptimal.

References

1. Lundberg S, Sodestrom J. Perforation of interventricular septum in myocardial infarction: a study based on autopsy material. *Acta Med Scand* 1962;172:413–42.
2. Terumi H, Sayuki K. Ventricular septal perforation with acute myocardial infarction. *Jpn Sci Technol* 2003;52:3083–90.
3. Kirklin JW, Barratt-Boyes BG. *Cardiac Surgery.* New York: John Wiley and Sons Inc. 6th edition. 1993. pp. 403–413.

20 Left Ventricular Mural Thrombus Following Myocardial Infarction

Xing Sheng Yang, Jing Ping Sun & Byron R. Williams Jr.
Emory University School of Medicine; Emory University Hospital Midtown, Atlanta, GA, USA

History

A 50-year-old male presented with breathing difficulty and chest pain. He has a history of drug abuse.

Physical Examination

Blood pressure (BP) was 172/127 mmHg, heart rate was 104/minute, and respiratory rate was 20/minute. Neck veins were distended. He had no significant heart murmur. Lungs revealed bibasilar rales.

Laboratory

Electrocardiogram showed flipped T waves in leads V5, aVF, and III, as well as peaked T waves in leads V2 and V3 symmetrically; a wide P wave in lead II was suggestive of atrial abnormality. Chest X-ray revealed cardiomegaly. His B natriuretic peptide was high at 2827.

Rest rubidium imaging demonstrated a dilated left ventricle (LV) cavity. There was an extensive defect involving the mid and basal portion of inferior and inferior septal walls. The defect was approximately 24% of the myocardium. Stress images showed a similar matched defect; this fixed defect suggested prior myocardial infarction.

Echocardiography demonstrated: (1) severely decreased LV and right ventricle systolic function; (2) moderately dilated LV; (3) akinetic and thinned inferior and inferoposterior wall; and (4) a mural LV thrombus along the anteroseptal wall. A long 1-cm-thick layered thrombus which was calcified covering the interventricular septum from base to apex in LV was noted (Figure 20.1 and Videoclip 20.1).

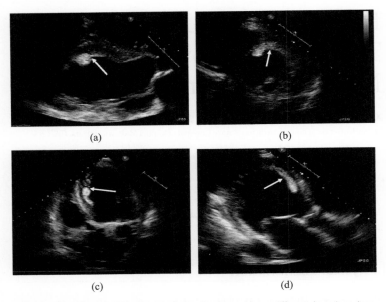

(a)   (b)

(c)   (d)

Figure 20.1. A ventricular septal mural thrombus (arrow) has a different shape in various views: (a) parasternal long-axis view; (b) parasternal short-axis view; (c) apical 4-chamber view; (d) apical long-axis view.

Discussion

The incidence of LV mural thrombi is higher in patients with anterior infarctions than in those with inferior infarctions [1]. Serial transthoracic echocardiography (TTE) study revealed most thrombi develop within the first 2 weeks after myocardial infarction [2]. However, some patients develop a new LV thrombus after discharge, often in association with worsening LV systolic function [3]. In our case, the mural thrombus was not in the myocardial infarction area, but this patient has a dilated LV with severely decreased systolic function and a history of drug abuse. The etiology of the cardiomyopathy may be both ischemic and nonischemic.

Several studies have shown that TTE has a sensitivity of 92–95% and a specificity approaching 95% for detecting LV thrombus, provided the echocardiographic image quality is adequate [4]. The site of attachment of the thrombus in the LV apex and its morphology could also be fully evaluated by live 3D TTE.

By using a higher frequency transducer, there will be less artifact introduced in most patients. Artifact can also be reduced by decreasing the focal zone to the depth of interest which can improve lateral resolution. A new thrombus may not be very echogenic and could be missed without a thorough echocardiographic examination.

References

1. Weinreich DJ, Burke JF, Pauletto FJ. Left ventricular mural thrombi complicating acute myocardial infarction long-term follow-up with serial echocardiography. *Ann Intern Med* 1984;100:789–94.
2. Nayak D, Aronow WS, Sukhija R, *et al.* Comparison of frequency of left ventricular thrombi in patients with anterior wall versus non-anterior wall acute myocardial infarction treated with antithrombotic and antiplatelet therapy with or without coronary revascularization. *Am J Cardiol* 2004;93:1529.
3. Greaves SC, Zhi G, Lee RT, *et al.* Incidence and natural history of left ventricular thrombus following anterior wall acute myocardial infarction. *Am J Cardiol* 1997;80:442.
4. Stratton JR, Lighty GW Jr, Pearlman AS, *et al.* Detection of left ventricular thrombus by two-dimensional echocardiography: sensitivity, specificity, and causes of uncertainty. *Circulation* 1982;66:156–66.

21 Inferior Wall Aneurysm Following Myocardial Infarction

Jing Ping Sun, Xing Sheng Yang & John D. Merlino

Emory University School of Medicine; Emory University Hospital Midtown, Atlanta, GA, USA

History

A 50-year-old male complains of chest pain with exertion. He was evaluated with a cardiac catheterization that showed multivessel coronary disease and inferior wall pseudoaneurysm. He was transferred to the hospital for surgical evaluation.

Physical Examination

Blood pressure was 148/92 mmHg; pulse was 92/minute. A 3/6 grade systolic ejection murmur was audible over the mitral valve area.

Laboratory

Echocardiogram: Left ventricle (LV) was severely dilated. The inferior wall appeared thin, and there was a huge inferior aneurysm at the base of the

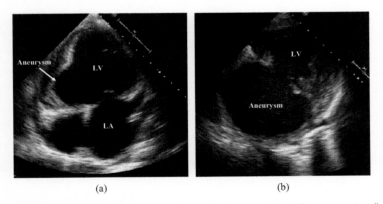

(a)   (b)

Figure 21.1. Transesophageal echocardiography: A large true ventricular aneurysm is well seen in this view (between 4- and 2-chamber views) (a). Parasternal short-axis view shows the large true basal posterior-septal and inferior wall aneurysm (b). LA, left atrium; LV, left ventricle.

Practical Handbook of Echocardiography 1st edition. Edited by Jing Ping Sun, Joel Felner and John Merlino. © 2010 Blackwell Publishing Ltd.

heart (Figure 21.1 and Videoclip 21.1). The LV EF was 15%. The basal, mid
of anteroseptal, and posterolateral basal walls were moderately
hypokinetic. The inferoposterior basal and septal basal walls were severely
hypokinetic (Videoclip 21.1). There was moderate mitral regurgitation and
thickened aortic valve leaflets.

Hospital Course

Patient underwent ventriculoplasty for a large inferior true aneurysm and
mitral repair by adjustment of the cordae. He was discharged on day 15
post operation in good condition.

Discussion

It was previously estimated that an LV aneurysm develops in up to 30–35%
of patients with Q wave MI [1]. However, the incidence of this
complication is decreasing, and currently is about 8 to 15 percent in such
patients [2]. This change is related to the introduction of major
improvements in the management of patients with acute myocardial
infarction (MI). Approximately 70–85% of LV aneurysms are located in
the anterior or apical walls due to total occlusion of the left anterior
descending coronary artery. Only 10–15% involve the inferior-basal walls
due to RCA occlusion.

The definition of true LV aneurysm is defined as an abnormal bulge in
the LV contour during both systole and diastole [3]. This definition
distinguishes aneurysms from dyskinetic segments in which the distortion
in shape presents only during systole. The wall of the aneurysm is typically
thin in comparison to the normal myocardium, and motion of the
aneurysmal segment is paradoxical. Comparable to the maximal diameter
of the true aneurysms, the diameter of the neck is wider.

In our case, the true aneurysm appears as a pseudoaneurysm in
individual view, the diameter of the neck is smaller than the maximal
diameter of the aneurysm in the parasternal short-axis view (Figure 21.1b).
It was diagnosed as an inferior wall pseudoaneurysm by another hospital,
indicating it is occasionally difficult to differentiate between true and
pseudoaneurysms. Review of multiple views is important for correct
diagnosis.

References

1. Mills NL, Everson CT, Hockmuth DR. Technical advances in the treatment of
   left ventricular aneurysm. *Ann Thorac Surg* 1993;55:792.
2. Nagle RE, Williams DO. Natural history of ventricular aneurysm without
   treatment. *Br Heart J* 1974;36:1037.
3. Weyman AE, Peskoe SM, Williams ES, *et al.* Detection of left ventricular
   aneurysm by cross-section echocardiography. *Circulation* 1976;54:936.

22 Isolated Right Ventricular Infarction

Jing Ping Sun, Xing Sheng Yang & John D. Merlino
Emory University School of Medicine; Emory University Hospital Midtown, Atlanta, GA, USA

History

A 60-year-old female complains of chest pain associated with nausea, diaphoresis, and shortness of breath.

Physical Examination

Temperature was 37.1°C, blood pressure was 147/73 mmHg, and the heart rate was 78 bpm. Patient's neck veins were distended. Cardiac auscultation was unremarkable.

Laboratory Study

Electrocardiogram revealed ST-segment elevations in leads that were consistent with an inferior distribution for infarct.

The coronary angiogram demonstrated no obstructive disease in the left coronary system, and a 95% ostial stenosis of a small nondominant right coronary artery (RCA).

Echocardiography: Mild concentric left ventricle hypertrophy and normal left ventricle (LV) chamber size. Left ventricle ejection fraction was 60%.

Right ventricle (RV) was severely dilated. Systolic function of the basal and mid segments of RV free wall was markedly reduced, but the contractility of the apex was preserved. The right atrium (RA) was dilated and the interatrial septum is bowed toward left atrium (LA) (Figure 22.1, Videoclip 22.1). The parasternal short-axis view showed that the LV was D-shaped during systole and diastole. (Figure 22.2, Videoclip 22.2).

Moderate TR with an RV estimated pressure of 34 mmHg was seen (Videoclip 22.3). Dilated IVC, with respiratory size variation greater than 50%, consistent with elevated RA pressure was noted. Trivial pericardial effusion was present.

Practical Handbook of Echocardiography 1st edition. Edited by Jing Ping Sun, Joel Felner and John Merlino. © 2010 Blackwell Publishing Ltd.

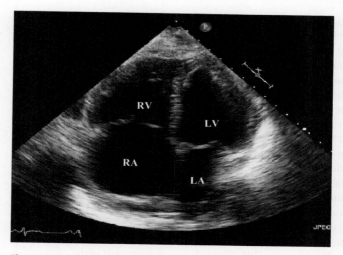

Figure 22.1. Apical 4-chamber view shows dilated right ventricle and right atrium. LA, left atrium; LV, left ventricle; RA, right atrium; RV, right ventricle.

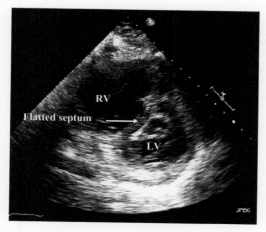

Figure 22.2. Parasternal short-axis view shows the flat septum. LV, left ventricle; RV, right ventricle.

Discussion

The RV has the same cardiac output as the LV. It has one-sixth as much muscle mass and performs one-fourth the stroke work, because the pulmonary vascular resistance is one-tenth of the systemic resistance [1].

The RCA supplies the RV lateral wall through the acute marginal branches. In the majority of patients, it also supplies the LV posterior wall and posterior interventricular septum through the posterior descending artery.

Infarction involving only RV and not LV is unusual. The reason appears to be that the prevalence of atherosclerosis in nondominant is less than in dominant RCAs [2]. In our case, coronary angiography revealed a 95% ostial stenosis of the nondominant RCA.

Echocardiography has become a useful tool in the diagnosis of right ventricular myocardial infarction (RVMI). Abnormal findings include RV dilatation, RV wall asynergy, and abnormal interventricular septal motion caused by a reversal of the transseptal pressure gradient due to the increased RV end-diastolic pressure. Interatrial septal bowing toward LA, indicative of an increased RA–LA pressure gradient, is an important prognostic marker in RVMI. All of these echocardiographic findings were present in our case.

High incidence of tricuspid regurgitation (TR) (such as in this case), and pericarditis is presumably due to the frequent transmural injury of the relatively thin-walled RV.

The strategy for the treatment of RVMI includes early maintenance of RV preload, reduction of RV afterload, inotropic support of the dysfunctional RV, and early reperfusion with fibrinolytic therapy or direct angioplasty.

References

1. Lee FA. Hemodynamics of the right ventricle in normal and diseased states. *Cardiol Clin* 1992;10:59–67.
2. Moreyra AE, Sclar C, Burns JJ, *et al.* Prevalence of angiographically recognizable atherosclerosis in non-dominant right coronary arteries. *Angiology* 1984;35:760–65.

23 Coronary Artery Fistula

Jing Ping Sun, Xing Sheng Yang, & John D. Merlino
Emory University School of Medicine; Emory University Hospital Midtown, Atlanta, GA, USA

History

Case 1 is a 41-year-old woman who complained of severe right infrascapular pain for 2–3 hours. The onset was abrupt and while at rest. There was no history of injury or strain. The pain was markedly worsened by deep breathing, and somewhat worsened also by movement of the shoulder and upper torso. It was located in the area just medial to the tip of her right scapula. She was short of breath. She has had no history of coronary disease or diabetes.

Case 2 is a 26-year-old female with end-stage renal disease and prolonged QT syndrome, and she has complained that her automatic implantable cardioverter defibrillator (AICD) fired once while at dialysis. Device interrogation demonstrated that the triggering event was an episode of atrial tachycardia. He adjusted the threshold for it to fire at a higher heart rate.

Physical Examination

In case 1, lungs are clear to auscultation, heart rate is regular, rhythm and S1, S2 were normal. No murmur was appreciated.

In case 2, there were no significantly findings on physical examination.

Laboratory Studies

Case 1: Results of catheterization shows that the aortic pressure was 190/110 (mean = 137). The left ventricular pressure was 190/20. The mean RA pressure was 5 ("a" wave = 9, "v" wave = 10). The right ventricular pressure was 38/5. The cardiac output was 7.32 L/min by Fick's principle. The systemic vascular resistance was 1497. The left and right coronaries were without evidence of atherosclerosis, but fistula from the distal left anterior descending (LAD) to the right ventricle (RV) was seen.

The subcostal 4-chamber view shows a color flow (arrow) away from RV apex, another coronary flow (long arrow) is well seen in RV apical wall; the flow (arrow) is clearly out of RV apex (Figure 23.1a,b and Videoclip 23.1a,b) in case 1. The apical 4-chamber (A4-ch) view shows that there is

Practical Handbook of Echocardiography 1st edition. Edited by Jing Ping Sun,
Joel Felner and John Merlino. © 2010 Blackwell Publishing Ltd.

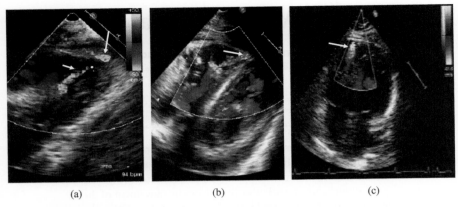

(a)   (b)   (c)

Figure 23.1. In case 1, the subcostal 4-chamber view shows a color flow (arrow) away from right ventricular apex, another coronary flow (long arrow) is well seen in right ventricular apical wall (a); this image shows that the flow (arrow) is clearly out of right ventricular apex (b). The apical 4-chamber view shows that there is an unusual color flow jet (arrow) near right ventricular apex in case 2 (c).

an unusual color flow jet near RV apex in case 2 (Figure 23.1c and Videoclip 23.1c).

The spectral Doppler recording from the unusual flow demonstrates a continuous flow during cardiac cycle, which suggests this is a coronary artery fistula into RV (Figure 23.2).

The color flows presented in diastole and systole suggest they are coronary artery fistulas into RV in both cases.

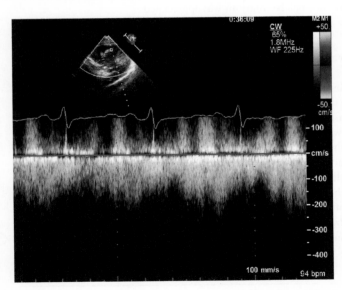

Figure 23.2. Spectral Doppler recording from the unusual flow demonstrates a continuous flow during cardiac cycle, which suggests this is a coronary artery fistula into right ventricle.

Discussion

Coronary artery fistula (CAF) accounts for 0.2–0.4% of congenital cardiac anomalies. Approximately 50% of pediatric coronary vasculature anomalies are CAFs [1]. Most CAF are congenital and may be found in patients with structurally normal hearts. Rarely, acquired forms of CAF may occur as a result of septal myectomy in association with hypertrophic cardiomyopathy, muscle bundle resection in operative repair of tetralogy of Fallot, as a complication of radiofrequency ablation of accessory pathways, penetrating or nonpenetrating trauma, endomyocardial biopsy, permanent pacemaker implantation, or as a complication of coronary arterial procedures [2]. A CAF involves a sizable communication between a coronary artery, bypasses the myocardial capillary bed, and enters either a chamber of the heart (coronary-cameral fistula) or any segment of the systemic or pulmonary circulation (coronary arteriovenous fistula). CAF can affect persons of any age. But Liberthson et al. [3] found that 91% of patients with these fistulas younger than 20 years were asymptomatic compared to 37% of patients older than 20 years. The symptoms or complications included congestive heart failure, myocardial ischemia, infective endocarditis, atrial fibrillation, pulmonary hypertension, and rupture. The pathophysiologic mechanism of CAF is myocardial stealing or reduction in myocardial blood flow distal to the site of the CAF connection with the fistula acting as a low resistance pathway. Diagnostic methods include physical examination, electrocardiography, chest X-ray, echocardiography, and angiocardiography.

In case 1 the patient had no history of coronary disease or diabetes. She has had no recent injury of any sort. The cardiac catherization indicated her coronary arteries were normal, except for a distal LAD to RV fistula. Almost certainly the fistula was congenital, and her chest pain was unrelated.

In case 2 the patient did have recent AICD, end-stage renal disease, and Methicillin-resistant Staphylococcus aureus bacteremia. This suggests the possibility of her coronary fistula having been mycotic, and secondary to coronary rupture as the result of infection. Another possibility is that the fistula may have been iatrogenic: possibly caused by guidewire perforation during the implantation of the cardioverter defibrillator.

Treatment: Spontaneous closure of a fistula is very uncommon. On the basis of these data, most authors have recommended surgical closure of these fistulas during childhood even in the absence of symptoms. The perioperative mortality rates ranged from 2 to 4 % in the literature.

In 1983, Reidy et al. [4] reported the first case of transcatheter embolization of a coronary artery fistula. Since then, several reports had demonstrated the feasibility of transcatheter closure of coronary artery fistulas. Coils, detachable balloons, umbrellas, and polyvinyl foam had been used for successful occlusion of these fistulas. The risks associated with transcatheter embolization of coronary artery fistulas include coronary artery disruption, pulmonary or systemic embolization, pericardial effusion, myocardial ischemia, or infarction. Recent results of both transcatheter and surgical approaches indicate a good prognosis. Approximately 4% of patients may require additional surgery for recurrence [5].

References

1. Carrel T, Tkebuchava T, Jenni R, *et al.* Congenital coronary fistulas in children and adults: diagnosis, surgical technique and results. *Cardiology* July–August 1996;87:325–30.
2. Said SA, el Gamal MI, van der Werf T. Coronary arteriovenous fistulas: collective review and management of six new cases – changing etiology, presentation, and treatment strategy. *Clin Cardiol* September 1997;20:748–52
3. Liberthson RR, Sagar K, Berkoben JP, *et al.* Congenital coronary arteriovenous fistula. Report of 13 patients, review of the literature and delineation of management. *Circulation* May 1979;59:849–54.
4. Reidy JF, Tynan MJ, Qureshi S. Embolisation of a complex coronary arteriovenous fistula in a 6 year old child: the need for specialised embolisation techniques. *Br Heart J* April 1990;63:246–8.
5. Trehan V, Yusuf J, Mukhopadhyay S, *et al.* Transcatheter closure of coronary artery fistulas. *Indian Heart J* March–April 2004;56:132–9.

24 Defined Location of Acute Myocardial Infarction by Two-D Strain Echocardiography Compared with Magnetic Resonance Imaging

Jing Ping Sun, Xing Sheng Yang, Robert D. O'Donnell Jr. & John D. Merlino

Emory University School of Medicine; Emory University Hospital Midtown, Atlanta, USA

History

A 70-year-old male was admitted with shortness of breath, associated chest tightness, and diaphoresis.

Physical Examination

The patient was in mild distress, tachycardic, and had a systolic heart murmur.

Laboratory

Catheterization revealed: a 100% mid-circumflex lesion, a 60–70% left anterior descending (LAD) lesion, and an occluded distal right coronary artery with collateral. Electrocardiogram (ECG) showed a right bundle branch block and Q waves in leads II, III and AVF.

Magnetic resonance imaging (MRI): The posterior and posterolateral walls of left ventricle (LV) were severely hypokinetic with edema.

Echocardiography

Transthoracic echocardiography showed mild left ventricular hypertrophy, and mildly decreased LV systolic function. The left atrial size was mildly

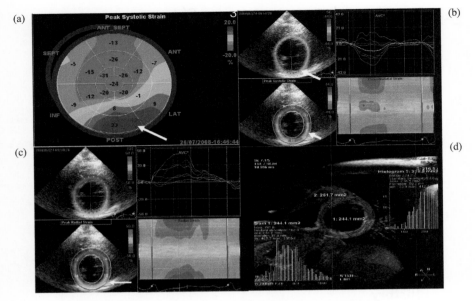

Figure 24.1. The bull's eye of two-dimensional longitudinal peak strain showed longitudinal was significantly reduced in the left ventricular posterior, postlateral wall (a). Circumferential (b) and radial (c) strain were reduced and the magnetic resonance image analysis showed edema (d) in the same area.

dilated. RV systolic function appeared normal. There was diastolic dysfunction in a pseudonormalization pattern. The LV inferoposterior and posterolateral walls were severely hypokinetic as demonstrated in parasternal long, apical 2-chamber, and apical long-axis views. Severe mitral regurgitation (MR) was noted (Videoclip 24.1). There was no pericardial effusion.

The two-dimensional (2D) strain image showed that the peak longitudinal, circumferential, and radial strain of the inferoposterior and posterolateral walls were significantly decreased (Figure 24.1, Videoclip 24.2). These results were consistent with the 2D image and the results of MRI, which indicated acute posterior and posterolateral wall infarction.

Discussion

Experimental studies have demonstrated that regional wall motion abnormalities can be visualized echocardiographically within 5–10 beats after coronary legation [1]. In these studies, functional changes can be observed to precede the development of ECG abnormalities. In clinical studies, stress-induced ischemia functional changes precede both ECG changes and pain.

This case showed typical regional wall motion abnormalities corresponding with the territory of 100% mid-circumflex coronary occlusion.

LV regional wall motion abnormalities during and immediately after myocardial infarction (MI) can lead to apical and posterior displacement of the papillary muscles with resulting malcoaptation of the mitral leaflets and mitral regurgitation [2].

The location and size of MI evaluated by 2D strain are consistent with the results of MRI in early damage of acute MI; which demonstrates that 2D strain can add data regarding LV segmental function, and defined location of acute MI.

References

1. Theroux P, Ross J Jr, Franklin D, Kemper WS, Sasyama S. Regional myocardial function in the conscious dog during acute coronary occlusion and response to morphine, propranolol, nitroglycerin and lidocacine. *Circulation* 1976;53:302.
2. Tcheng JE, Jackman JD Jr, Nelson CL, *et al.* Outcome of patients sustaining acute ischaemic mitral regurgitation during myocardial infarction. *Ann Intern Med* 1992;117:18–24.

Part 6
Pulmonary Artery Diseases

25 Pulmonary Embolism

Jing Ping Sun, Seth Clemens & John D. Merlino

Emory University School of Medicine; Emory University Hospital Midtown, Atlanta, GA, USA

Case Report

A 48-year-old male presented with increasing shortness of breath and dry cough for 5 days. The patient had an 8-year history of cocaine abuse and positive HIV.

Physical Examination

Blood pressure was 121/90 mmHg, heart rate was 137/minute, respiratory rate was 20/minute. Heart: regular rate without murmurs or gallop. Lungs were clear.

Echcardiography: The left ventricle (LV) size and systolic function are normal. There is mild left ventricular hypertrophy. The right ventricle (RV) is severely dilated with mildly hypertrophied wall, and there is severe hypokinesis in RV basal and middle segments. RV apical contractility was preserved (McConnell's sign). A D-shaped septum was noted in both systole and diastole consistent with RV pressure overload (Figure 25.1, Videoclip 25.1). Moderate tricuspid regurgitation (TR) is present. The TR velocity is 2.76 m/sec with estimated RV systolic pressure is moderately elevated at 50.5 mmHg.

RV dysfunction was further confirmed by tissue Doppler image analysis (Figure 25.2).

Initial electrocardiogram showed sinus tachycardia with very mild ST elevation in leads V1 and V2.

Computed tomography scan of the chest revealed bilateral upper and lower lobe pulmonary emboli (Figure 25.3).

The patient underwent inferior vena cava filter placement and was initiated on anticoagulation.

Discussion

Several echocardiographic findings have been proposed for noninvasive diagnosis of RV dysfunction due to pulmonary embolism (PE), including RV enlargement and/or hypokinesis of the free wall, leftward septal shift, and evidence of pulmonary hypertension [1]. The quantitative measurements for supporting the PE diagnosis include (1) RV end

Practical Handbook of Echocardiography 1st edition. Edited by Jing Ping Sun, Joel Felner and John Merlino. © 2010 Blackwell Publishing Ltd.

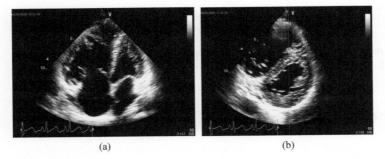

(a)   (b)

Figure 25.1. The right ventricle is severely dilated with mildly hypertrophied wall (a), a flat septum was noted in parasternal short-axis view (b).

diastolic (ED) diameter > 25 mm; (2) RVED/LVED diameter ratio >0.5; (3) RVED/LVED area ratio >0.6; (4) estimated systolic pulmonary artery pressure >35 mmHg. All of the echocardiographic findings above were detected in our case.

Preservation of RV apical function relative to the RV free wall function, McConell's sign [1], suggests PE as an etiology of RV dysfunction. The tissue Doppler of RV free wall was analyzed in our case; the results were consistent with RV free wall dysfunction. The data of Tissue Doppler imaging

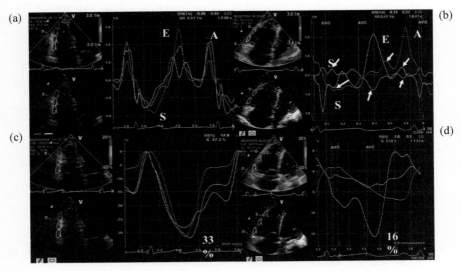

Figure 25.2. The longitudinal strain rate of right ventricular segments from a normal person (a). The longitudinal strain rate is decreased and desynchronized in a patient with pulmonary embolism (b). The peak of longitudinal segment strain is 33% and synchronized from a normal person (c). The peak of longitudinal segment strain is decreased and desynchronized (d) in our case.

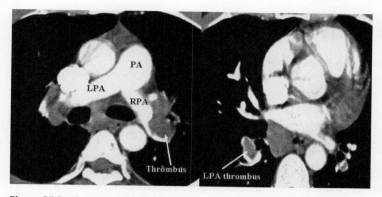

Figure 25.3. The computed tomography scan of the chest revealed bilateral upper and lower lobe pulmonary emboli. PA, pulmonary artery; LPA, left pulmonary artery; RPA, right pulmonary artery.

added more information in diagnosis of pulmonary embolism, which may add to the clinical utility of echocardiography in patients with PE.

Reference

1. McConnell MV, Solomon SD, Rayan ME, Come PC, Goldhaber SZ, Lee RT. Regional right ventricular dysfunction detected by echocardiography in acute pulmonary embolism. *Am J Cardiol* 1996;78(4): 469–73.

26 Pulmonary Emboli

Dale Yoo & Jing Ping Sun

Emory University School of Medicine; Emory University Hospital Midtown, Atlanta, GA, USA

Studied Cases

Case 1: A 32-year-old male with sudden onset chest pain and shortness of breath. Transthoracic echocardiography (TTE) revealed normal left ventricle (LV) function and size, but was significant for a large right ventricle–right atrium (RV–RA) gradient of 84 mmHg as well as a severely hypokinetic RV. Upon further examination, a large pulmonary saddle embolus was visualized in the main pulmonary, which almost occluded the left main pulmonary artery (PA) and partially occluded the right PA as well (Figure 26.1, Videoclip 26.1a,b). He had borderline hypotension. The patient was taken to the interventional laboratory and given directed tPA which did not decrease the size of the embolus. Nonetheless, the patient remained stable and normotensive with a 250-mL bolus of normal saline and initiation of a dopamine drip. Coumadin was initiated.

Case 2: A 83-year-old male with recurrent dizziness and acute renal failure. During the admission, he became unresponsive and acutely short of breath which resulted in an emergent intubation and mechanical ventilation. A TTE revealed normal LV systolic function; RV and IVC were dilated. Transesophageal echocardiography showed a large embolus in the main PA (Videoclip 26.1 c,d). The PA systolic pressure was 55 mmHg.

Discussion

Acute pulmonary embolism (PE) is a common condition that often results in fatal outcomes. Strictly defined, PE is an obstruction of the pulmonary arterial vasculature by materials including but not limited to air, tumor, fat, and thrombus [1]. PE is the consequence of these materials dislodging from other locations of the body and moving into the lungs.

We report two cases of PE, one of a saddle PE in an otherwise healthy patient and another with acute renal failure.

The management of PE almost always begins with the initiation of an anticoagulant, such as heparin. Although it does not actively serve as a thrombolytic, it prevents further thrombus formation. The use of a thrombolytic is usually reserved for severely decompensated patients with cardiogenic shock and hypotension, when the diagnosis is highly probable for PE. The evidence for its benefit is also questionable.

Practical Handbook of Echocardiography 1st edition. Edited by Jing Ping Sun, Joel Felner and John Merlino. © 2010 Blackwell Publishing Ltd.

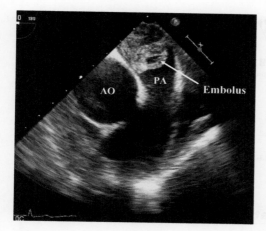

Figure 26.1. Transthoracic echocardiography: parasternal short-axis view shows a large embolus (arrow) in the main pulmonary. AO, aorta; PA, pulmonary artery.

Given the difficulty of initial diagnosis based on clinical data, a computed tomography specific for PE will be done first, as long as the renal function permits. TTE is often performed to better elucidate a possible thrombus as well as determine left and right cardiac function and size. RV–RA gradient and a PA pressure can be estimated based on echocardiographic data. In our cases above, the acute PE led to elevation of right-sided pressures in addition to RV hypokinesis due to pressure and volume overload. The TTE data can assist the clinician in determining the need for inotropic agents as well as intravenous fluid, which is most valuable in the critically ill patients with massive PE [2].

References

1. Goldhaber SZ. Pulmonary embolism. *N Engl J Med* 1998;339:93–104.
2. Sadosty AT, Boie ET, Stead LG. Pulmonary embolism. *Emerg Med Clin North Am* 2003;21:363–84.

27 Pulmonary Artery Dissection

Xiaofang Lu & Xin-Fang Wang

Huazhong University of Science and Technology; Union Hospital of HUST, Wuhan, Hubei, China

History

A 20-year-old male has had palpitations and shortness of breath for the past 10 days.

Physical Examination

Temperature was 36.8°C, heart rate was 140/minute, blood pressure was 130/50 mmHg, and respiration rate of 26/minute. Cyanosis of lips was found. Cardiac examination revealed regular tachycardia, auscultation found a loud pulmonary component of S2, there was a 4/6 continuous murmur along the upper left sternal border and a 3/5 systolic murmur in sub-xyphoid area.

Laboratory

Chest X-ray revealed pulmonary artery (PA), left atrium, and left ventricle (LV) enlargement.

Electrocardiogram revealed tachycardia, atrial fibrillation, and global ST-segment depression. Echocardiography: LV and RV chambers were enlarged. The main trunk, left and right branches of the pulmonary artery were dilated. A dissected intimal flap was noted in the main pulmonary trunk originating from 1.3 cm above the pulmonary valve and extending to the bifurcation (Figure 27.1, Videoclip 27.1). Severe pulmonary valve insufficiency and mild TR were detected. Pulmonary systolic pressure estimated by the pressure gradient across tricuspid valve was 90 mmHg. A patent duct artery (PDA) channel was detected. Color Doppler showed that the shunt of PDA ran into the true lumen of PA (Videoclip 27.2b).

Magnetic resonance imaging confirmed the presence of PA dissection and PDA.

Management

Closure of PDA and aneurysmorrhaphy of PA dissection was performed at surgery.

Practical Handbook of Echocardiography 1st edition. Edited by Jing Ping Sun, Joel Felner and John Merlino. © 2010 Blackwell Publishing Ltd.

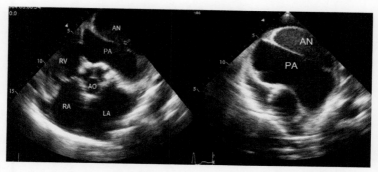

Figure 27.1. Parasternal short axis views show intimal flap in the main pulmonary trunk and formed pulmonary artery dissection. AN, aneurysm; AO, aorta; LA, left atrium; PA, pulmonary artery; RA, right atrium; RV, right ventricle.

Discussion

Pulmonary artery dissection is a rare but life-threatening event. It always occurs in patients with pulmonary hypertension of various causes, and at the site of anueysm or dilation of PA. The most frequent cause is a congenital cardiovascular anomaly, with PDA as the most common [1]. It is assumed that pulmonary hypertension resulting in mucoid degeneration of the media and fragmentation of the elastic fibers predispose to this condition. Although rare, PA dissection has been reported in patients without underlying pulmonary hypertension, such as connective tissue disease, chronic inflammation, etc. [2].

The main pulmonary trunk is the site of dissection in most patients, usually without involvement of the branches. The remainder of the sites are isolated right or left PAs and intrapulmonary branches.

The false lumen of PA dissection tends to rupture rather than to develop a re-entry site, as is usual in aortic dissection, leading to sudden death. Rupture occurs most commonly into surrounding organs and tissues, the pericardium, rarely the lungs, mediastinum and pleural cavity.

The clinical symptoms of PA dissection are generally nonspecific, usually exertional dyspnea, retrosternal chest pain, and central cyanosis. This makes it difficult to diagnose clinically. With the development of noninvasive cardiac imaging modalities, more PA dissection has been diagnosed during life.

References

1. Khattar RS, Fox DJ, Alty JE, *et al.* Pulmonary artery dissection: an emerging cardiovascular complication in surviving patients with chronic pulmonary hypertension. *Heart* 2005 February;91(2):142–5.
2. Inayama Y, Nakatani Y, Kitamura H. Pulmonary artery dissection in patients without underlying pulmonary hypertension. *Histopathology* 2001 May;38(5):435–42.

Part 7
Congenital Heart Disease

28 Unicuspid Aortic Valve

Jing Ping Sun[1], Xing Sheng Yang[1] & James D. Thomas[2]

[1] Emory University School of Medicine; Emory University Hospital Midtown, Atlanta, GA, USA
[2] The Cleveland Clinic Foundation, Cleveland, OH, USA

History

A 40-year-old man presents with 3 days history of intermittent, escalating dyspnea and chest tightness. As a child, he was told that he had a precordial murmur.

Physical Examination

Respiratory rate was 32/minute, heart rate was 110/minute, and blood pressure was 148/90 mmHg. Cardiac examination revealed a regular cardiac rate, a 4/6 systolic murmur heard best at the right upper sternal border.

Laboratory

Transesophageal echocardiography (TEE) revealed an anatomical unicuspid aortic valve and systolic doming (Figure 28.1). The peak gradient is 60.0 and mean gradient is 27.0 mmHg. There is severe prolapse of the aortic cusp(s) with 2+ to 3+ aortic regurgitation with eccentric directed posteriorly jet (Videoclip 28.1).

Discussion

Unicuspid aortic valve (UAV) is a rare congenital malformation seen in approximately 0.02% of patients referred for echocardiography but in as many as 4% to 6% of patients undergoing operations for "pure aortic stenosis" [1]. In early adulthood, degenerative fibrosis and calcification result in aortic stenosis and, less commonly, regurgitation. This case has UAV with 2+ to 3+ aortic regurgitation eccentric directed posteriorly. UAV is often confused with a bicuspid valve. The symptomatology between unicuspid and bicuspid aortic valves remains indistinguishable. Syncope, angina, and shortness of breath are common manifestations of outflow obstructive lesions, which include bicuspid and unicuspid aortic valves, subaortic membranes, and idiopathic HCM. TEE is an effective diagnostic

Practical Handbook of Echocardiography 1st edition. Edited by Jing Ping Sun,
Joel Felner and John Merlino. © 2010 Blackwell Publishing Ltd.

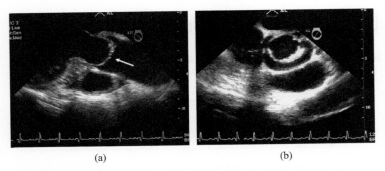

(a)   (b)

Figure 28.1. Transesophageal echocardiogram images illustrate: (a) systolic doming (arrow), (b) a unicuspid unicommissural valve.

tool to distinguish among these abnormalities [2]. Two forms of UAV have been recognized: the acommissural and the unicommissural, the latter predominates in both adult and pediatric populations [1]. The acommissural form has a single membrane-like leaflet with a central stenotic orifice and no lateral attachment to the aorta. The unicommissural type is the most common form and has one lateral attachment to the aorta and two raphes where the leaflets should have formed, resulting in an orifice shaped like an exclamation mark when viewed from above. Both configurations have a dome shape.

The regurgitant unicuspid aortic valve can be repaired successfully and reproducibly by converting it into bicuspid anatomy. The functional results are comparable with those obtained in reconstructed bicuspid aortic valves. With this approach, replacement can be avoided in most patients [3].

References

1. Agnihotri AK, Desai SC, Lai YQ, *et al.* Two distinct clinical presentations in adult unicuspid aortic valve. *J Thorac Cardiovasc Surg* 2006;131:1169–70.
2. Espinal M, Fuisz AR, Nanda NC, *et al.* Sensitivity and specificity of transesophageal echocardiography for determination of aortic valve morphology. *Am Heart J* 2000;139:1071–76.
3. Hans-Joachim S, Diana A, Svetlana R, *et al.* Bicuspidization of the unicuspid aortic valve: a new reconstructive approach. *Ann Thorac Surg* 2008;85:2012–8.

29 Bicuspid Aortic Valve

Xing Sheng Yang[1], Jing Ping Sun[1] & Joel M. Felner[2]
[1]Emory University School of Medicine; Emory Hospital Midtown, Atlanta, GA, USA
[2]Grady Memorial Hospital; Emory University School of Medicine, Atlanta, GA, USA

History

Patients with bicuspid aortic valves may be completely asymptomatic. If symptoms present, they relate to the development of aortic stenosis, insufficiency, or both.

Physical Examination

Bicuspid aortic valve is frequently a clinically silent condition; general examination findings may be normal. The most common abnormal sound heard with bicuspid aortic valve is a systolic ejection click. It is heard in all phases of respiration just after the first heart sound, and its timing does not vary with maneuvers (e.g., hand-grip, Valsalva, squatting).

Laboratory

Echocardiography: Abnormal eccentric coaptation line, systolic leaflet doming and abnormal pattern of systolic opening are observed in parasternal long and short-axis views as well as M-mode echocardiography. A series of echocardiographic recordings from 6 patients with different types of bicuspid aortic valves is illustrated (Figures 29.1–29.3, Videoclips 29.1 and 29.2).

Discussion

Bicuspid valves are clinically important because they can be associated with significant aortic valve stenosis (AS), reflecting the propensity for premature fibrosis, stiffening, and calcium deposition [1]. Bicuspid valves frequently cause aortic regurgitation (AR), are associated with aortic root dilation, are a site for endocarditis, and may be associated with other congenital cardiac abnormalities.

Serial assessment of the aortic valve by echocardiography is a valuable tool to evaluate the function of the valve as well as to measure the aortic diameter, left ventricular chamber dimensions, and ventricular function

Practical Handbook of Echocardiography 1st edition. Edited by Jing Ping Sun, Joel Felner and John Merlino. © 2010 Blackwell Publishing Ltd.

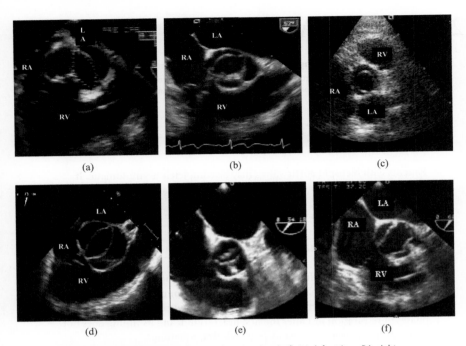

Figure 29.1. Different types of bicuspid aortic valves (a–f). LA, left atrium; RA, right atrium; RV, right ventricle.

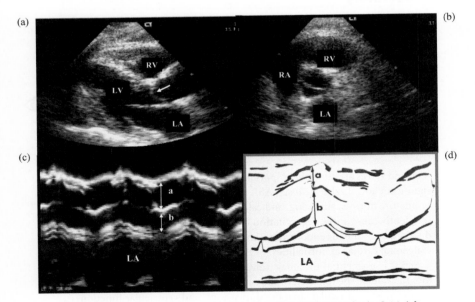

Figure 29.2. Images illustrate eccentric closing line of bicuspid aortic valve (a–d). LA, left atrium; LV, left ventricle; RA, right atrium; RV, right ventricle.

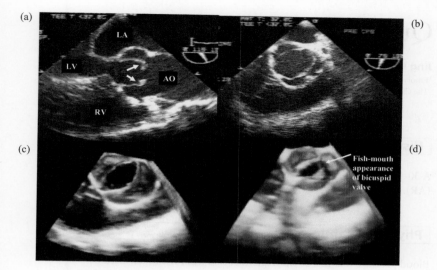

Figure 29.3. (a–d) Two-dimensional and three-dimensional images from parasternal window illustrate the different bicuspid aortic valves. AO, aorta; LA, left atrium; LV, left ventricle; RV, right ventricle.

[2]. The echocardiographic diagnosis is based on the demonstration of two cusps and two commissures during direct short-axis recording. In long axis, an abnormal or eccentric coaptation line may be seen along with systolic leaflet doming and an abnormal pattern of systolic opening. However, echocardiographic identification of a bicuspid aortic valve can be obscured in severe stenosis and after cuspal fusion secondary to inflammation.

Patients with bicuspid aortic valve were previously advised to take antibiotic prophylaxis. Since the revised AHA guidelines in 2007, antibiotic prophylaxis is no longer advocated before dental and other procedures. The indications for percutaneous or surgical intervention are the same as for patients with AR or AS for any cause [3].

References

1. Fedak PWM, Verma S, David TE, *et al.* Clinical and pathophysiological implications of a bicuspid aortic valve. *Circulation* 2002;106:900–905.
2. Burks JM, Illes RW, Keating EC, *et al.* Ascending aortic aneurysm and dissection in young adults with bicuspid aortic valve: implications for echocardiographic surveillance. *Clin Cardiol* 1998;21:439–43.
3. David T Ei. Surgical treatment of aortic valve endocarditis. In: Cohn LH, ed. *Cardiac Surgery in the Adult.* New York: McGraw-Hill, 2008. pp. 949–56.

30 Quadricuspid Aortic Valve

Jing Ping Sun[1], Xing Sheng Yang[1] & James D. Thomas[2]

[1] Emory University School of Medicine; Emory University Hospital Midtown, Atlanta, GA, USA
[2] The Cleveland Clinic Foundation, Cleveland, OH, USA

History

A 30-year-old male presented with a 5-year history of aortic regurgitation (AR).

Physical Examination

Blood pressure was 124/60 mmHg; heart rate was 71/minute. Cardiac exam revealed a diastolic murmur consistent with AR.

Laboratory

Echocardiography: Quadricuspid aortic valve was seen in the parasternal short-axis view, which corresponds with surgical field (Figure 30.1, Videoclip 30.1). There was AR with anteriorly directed jet, vena contracta 0.73 cm (Videoclip 30.1). Left ventricle (LV) was mildly dilated with mild systolic dysfunction.

Computed tomography scan suggested that the aortic diameter was relatively normal and that the descending aorta was entirely normal.

Coronary arteriogram documented normal coronary arteries.

Because the patient had moderate AR and LV dysfunction, to avoid irreversible myocardial dysfunction, the patient underwent aortic valve replacement with a #27–29 On-X mechanical bileaflet prosthesis and reduction aortoplasty (plication between felt strips).

Discussion

Quadricuspid aortic valve is a rare anomaly with a reported incidence of between 1 in 2500 and 1 in 10000 in autopsy studies [1]. A modern echocardiography database review showed the prevalence to be somewhat higher, from 0.013 to 0.043% depending on the years reviewed [2]. Valve replacement is frequently required in the fifth or sixth decade of life [3]. Aortic valve surgery is indicated in symptomatic patients and recommended in asymptomatic patients with evidence of LV systolic

Practical Handbook of Echocardiography 1st edition. Edited by Jing Ping Sun, Joel Felner and John Merlino. © 2010 Blackwell Publishing Ltd.

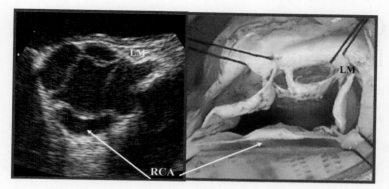

Figure 30.1. Congenital quadricuspid aortic valve echo-anatomic correlation. LM, left main coronary artery; RCA, right coronary artery.

dysfunction (LV ejection fraction <50%) or LV enlargement (LV end-systolic dimension >55 mm, or LV end-diastolic dimension >75 mm), such as the present case, who has not yet progressed to the decompensated stage [4].

References

1. Hurwitz LE, Roters WC. Quadricuspid semilunia valves. *Am J Cardiol* 1973;31(5):623–26.
2. Feldman BJ, Khandheria BK, Warnes CA, *et al.* Incidence, description and functional assessment of isolated quadricuspid aortic valves. *Am J Cardiol* 1990;65:937–8.
3. Timperley J, Milner R, Marshall AJ, Gilbert TJ. Quadricuspid aortic valves. *Clin Cardiol* 2002;25:548–52.
4. Brzezinski M, Mertz V, Clements FM. Transesophageal echocardiography of the quadricuspid aortic valve. *Anesth Analg* 2006;103:1414–15.

31 Congenital Left Ventricular Diverticulum

Yunhua Gao[1], Yali Xu[1] & Xing Sheng Yang[2]

[1] The Third Military Medical University; XinQiao Hospital, ChongQing, China
[2] Emory University School of Medicine; Emory University Hospital Midtown, Atlanta, GA, USA

History

A 4-year-old girl was found to have a pulsating mass of the abdominal wall since birth.

Physical Examination

Pulsating mass was found at abdominal region just superior to the umbilicus. Pulsation of the mass coincided with the heartbeat. Systolic and diastolic murmurs were heard upon auscultation of the mass.

Laboratory

Echocardiography demonstrated a pulsating tubular image running along with the mass (Figure 31.1). The mass appeared to be connected with the cardiac apex and terminated distally at a blind end at the umbilical level. The diameter of the blind end was 9.3 mm. The narrowest region was 2.5 mm with a wall thickness of 4 mm. Color Doppler showed a mosaic blue-red turbulent flow pattern in the tubule from the cardiac apex (Figure 31.2). Pulsed wave spectral Doppler revealed a pulsatile pattern of antegrade and retrograde flow with a maximum antegrade velocity of 174 cm/sec (Figure 31.3). Echocardiography revealed dextrocardia without ventricular or septal defects. Imaging with digital subtraction contrast angiography revealed a mass on the superior abdominal wall communicating with the left ventricle (LV) apex.

The diagnosis of an LV diverticulum terminating in the superior abdominal wall was confirmed by surgical and pathological findings.

Discussion

Congenital LV diverticulum is a rare cardiac malformation. Its incidence is approximately 0.4% in autopsies of patients expiring from cardiac disease,

Practical Handbook of Echocardiography 1st edition. Edited by Jing Ping Sun,
Joel Felner and John Merlino. © 2010 Blackwell Publishing Ltd.

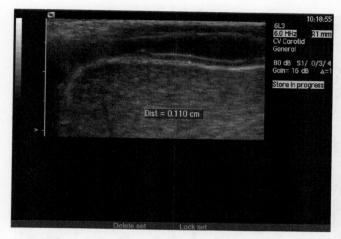

Figure 31.1. Two-dimensional echocardiography demonstrating a pulsating tubular structure on the superior abdominal wall.

and in approximately 0.26% in nonselected patients undergoing cardiac catheterization [1]. It appears to be a developmental anomaly, starting in the fourth embryonic week, and can be explained by a partial stop in the development of the embryonic ventricle [2]. A typical congenital cardiac diverticulum is characterized by a finger-like projection emerging from LV wall, contracting in synchrony with the corresponding chamber. The communication to the ventricular cavity is narrow and tubular. Diagnosis can be established by echocardiography, magnetic resonance imaging, or LV angiography. Some authors have advocated surgical revision in all cases

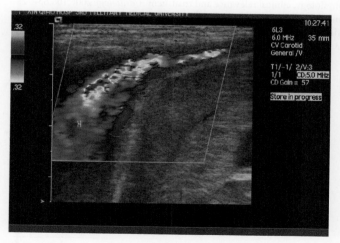

Figure 31.2. Color flow Doppler demonstrates blood flow arising from the apex of left ventricle.

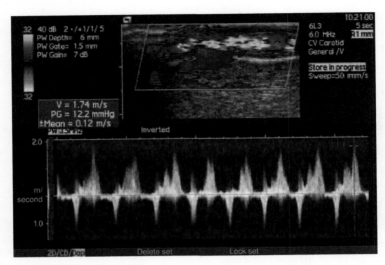

Figure 31.3. Pulsed wave spectral Doppler demonstrates antegrade and retrograde flow.

of diverticulum due to the presence of or potential for thrombus leading to embolism and/or the development of cardiac dysrhythmias [3]. However, due to the lack of larger trials with longer observation periods, no firm consensus has been reached with respect to optimal management.

References

1. Makaryus AN, Peters MR. Clinical images: congenital left ventricular diverticulum diagnosed by 64-detector CT imaging. *J Invasive Cardiol* 2008;20:372–3.
2. Ohlow MA. Congenital left ventricular aneurysms and diverticula: definition, pathophysiology, clinical relevance and treatment. *Cardiology* 2006;106:63–72.
3. Pradhan M, Dalal A, Kappor A, *et al.* Fetal left ventricular diverticulum presenting as dysrhythmia: diagnosis and management. *Fetal Diagn Ther* 2008;23:10–14.

32 Congenital Abnormality of the Mitral Valve Apparatus

Robert C. Bahler

Case Western University; Heart and Vascular Center, MetroHealth Medical Center, Cleveland, OH, USA

Shone's complex and the associated parachute mitral valve (MV) have been described predominantly in infants and children [1]. The structural alterations of the MV complex may be accompanied by a supramitral ring, a hypoplastic aortic arch, coarctation of the aorta, and aortic valve (AV) abnormalities.

A 35-year-old man presented with palpitations but otherwise asymptomatic. Echocardiographic images demonstrated an abnormal MV with a prominent papillary muscle that narrowed left ventricular outflow tract (LVOT) during systole (Figure 32.1). Proximal flow convergence in mid- left ventricle (mid-LV) confirmed the site of LVOT obstruction (Figure 32.2, Videoclip 32.1). The LVOT gradient was 12 mmHg. Mitral valve stenosis (MS) and mitral regurgitation (MR) were present (Figure 32.3). The AV and aorta were normal. The systolic pulmonary artery pressure was 37 mmHg.

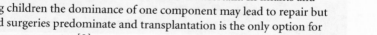

Exercise echocardiography: The patient achieved 10 metabolic equivalent tasks (METs) of exercise but blood pressure fell to 86/50 mmHg at peak stress. The echocardiographic imaging began 15 seconds after exercise ended and revealed an MS gradient of 33 mmHg, a systolic gradient between LV and left atrium (LA) of 196 mmHg and an LVOT gradient of 150 mmHg. Assuming the arterial systolic pressure was still around 86 mmHg at the time of these images, the LV systolic pressure below LVOT would be 236 mmHg. It is likely that LA pressure at this time point approximates 40 mmHg resulting in an LV–LA gradient of around 190 mmHg (Figure 32.4). These marked hemodynamic alterations with exercise illustrate the complexity of the congenital abnormality.

Management of this condition in adults is uncertain. In infants and young children the dominance of one component may lead to repair but staged surgeries predominate and transplantation is the only option for perhaps one-quarter [2].

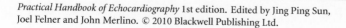

Practical Handbook of Echocardiography 1st edition. Edited by Jing Ping Sun, Joel Felner and John Merlino. © 2010 Blackwell Publishing Ltd.

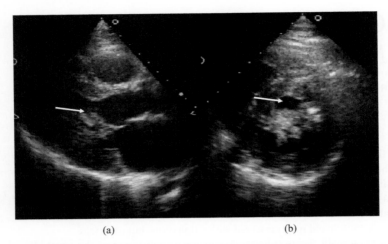

(a)   (b)

Figure 32.1. Large papillary muscle impinging on the left ventricular septum (arrow) during systole and a structurally abnormal mitral valve are seen both in the (PSL) (a) and parasternal short-axis (b) views. Thickening of the mitral valve leaflets is evident.

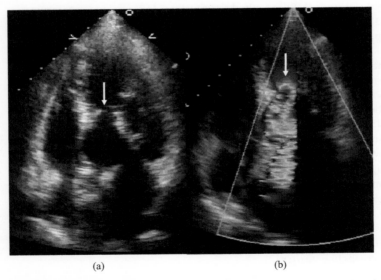

(a)   (b)

Figure 32.2. Apical 4-chamber view clarifies the location of the large papillary muscle and its proximity to the left ventricle septum. Note that the mitral valve stenosis obstruction (arrow) is located more towards the mid-left ventricle as compared to rheumatic mitral valve stenosis (a). Systolic color flow convergence (arrow) develops at the mid-left ventricle below the left ventricle outflow obstruction. Mitral regurgitation is evident but a significant portion of the regurgitant jet is shadowed by the large papillary muscle (b).

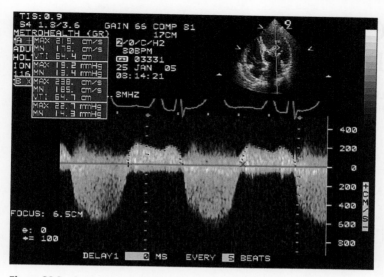

Figure 32.3. Continuous wave Doppler of mitral flow demonstrates both mitral regurgitation with a left ventricle–left atrium gradient of 140 mmHg and mitral valve stenosis with a mean gradient of 14 mmHg.

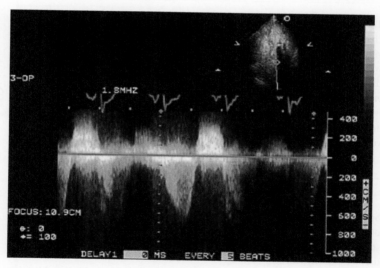

Figure 32.4. Mitral valve stenosis mean gradient is 30–35 mmHg. The contour of systolic velocities is consistent with left ventricular outflow obstruction with a peak gradient of 150 mmHg. The first and third complexes of this frame include part of the mitral regurgitation velocity profile with a peak left ventricle–left atrium gradient of approximately 196 mmHg.

References

1. Ikemba CM, Eidem BW, Fraley K, *et al.* Mitral valve morphology and morbidity/mortality in Shone's complex. *Am J Cardiol* 2005;95:541–3.
2. Prunier F, Furber AP, Laporte J, Geslin P. Discovery of a parachute mitral valve complex (Shone's anomaly) in an adult. *Echocardiograpy* 2001;18:179–82.

33 Congenital Left Ventricular Diverticulum

Lin He, Xin-Fang Wang & Ming Xing Xie

Huazhong University of Science and Technology; Union Hospital of HUST, Wuhan, Hubei, China

History

A 4-year-old boy was admitted for evaluation of syncope.

Physical Examination

The cardiac physical exam was normal.

Laboratory

Transthoracic echocardiography demonstrated a large cystic accessory chamber arising from the intersection of the mitral valve and the aortic valve ring between the ascending aorta and left atrium. It communicated with the main left ventricle (LV) chamber through an orifice (1.8 cm in diameter). The wall was thin and smooth. Diverticular chamber was enlarged in systole (Figure 33.1, Videoclip 33.1). LV was mildly dilated with normal contraction. Color Doppler imaging demonstrated flow into and out of the diverticulum. Surgery demonstrated a congenital left ventricular diverticulum (LVD).

Discussion

Secondary LVD may be due to: (1) excessive increase of LV pressure occurring in idiopathic hypertrophic subaortic stenosis, and aortic valve stenosis; (2) local thinning of the wall of LV occurring in ischemic heart disease and myocarditis [1].

Congenital diverticula can be associated with a congenital isolated local reduction of cardiac muscle fibers or fibrous tissue replacement of myocardium. The area of the myocardial deficiency may expand and result in the formation of LVD by high LV pressure. There are two types of congenital LVD: fibrous and muscular: (1) muscular diverticula are usually located in the apex, and generally communicate with the main LV chamber through a narrow orifice. They may appear cystic or hemispheric. Muscular

Practical Handbook of Echocardiography 1st edition. Edited by Jing Ping Sun, Joel Felner and John Merlino. © 2010 Blackwell Publishing Ltd.

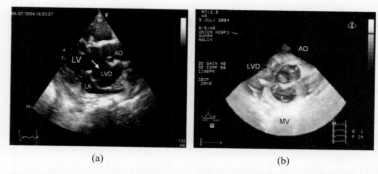

(a)   (b)

Figure 33.1. Diverticulum communicates with the main left ventricle chamber through an orifice (a). Three-dimensional image showed the diverticulum between ascending aorta and left atrium (b). AO, aorta; LA, left atrium; LV, left ventricle; LVD, left ventricular diverticulum; MV, mitral valve.

diverticula may often be partially contractile and synchronous with the contraction of the main chamber. Patients with muscular diverticula often have other abnormalities such as Cantrell syndrome; (2) Fibrous diverticula occur less frequently than muscular LVD and are usually located at the fibrous ring between the mitral and aortic valves. Secondary aortic valvular stenosis or regurgitation has been described. Fibrous diverticula have no contractile function, and generally occur in isolation without other abnormalities. The patient can be asymptomatic [2,3].

References

1. Okereke OUI, Cooley DA, Frazier OH. Congenital diverticulum of the ventricle. *J Thorac Cardiovasc Surg* 1986;91:208.
2. Head HD, Jue KL, Askren CC. Aortic subannular ventricular aneurysm. *Ann Thorac Surg* 1993;55:1268.
3. Teske DW, McGovern JJ, Allen HD. Congenital fibrous left ventricular diverticulum. *Am Heart J* 1993;126:1233.

34 Supracristal Ventricular Septal Defect

Jing Ping Sun, Robert D. O'Donnell Jr. & John D. Merlion
Emory University School of Medicine; Emory University Hospital Midtown, Atlanta, GA, USA

History

A 50-year-old female diagnosed with a small atrial septal defect since childhood.

Physical Examination

Blood pressure was 134/83 mmHg; heart rate was 70 and regular. The cardiac exam revealed a short systolic murmur.

Laboratory

Electrocardiogram showed nonspecific ST-segment abnormalities, but with no sign of right ventricular enlargement or hypertrophy.

Echocardiography: Both atria and ventricles were normal in size and function. There was normal valvular function. A small infundibular subarterial ventricular septal defect (VSD) was detected by color Doppler in apical 4-chamber and parasternal long-axis views (Figure 34.1a). The shunt was seen in the magnetic resonance images (arrow pointed in Figure 34.2), it was just below the aortic valve on two-dimensional and three-dimensional echocardiographic images (Videoclips 34.1 and 34.2).

The patient's shunt is hemodynamically insignificant and is unlikely to cause symptoms or progress.

Discussion

There are various types of VSD; the infundibular ventriculoseptal-type occurs less frequently representing 5–7% of VSDs [1]. This type of septal defect is located under both semilunar valves, at the fibrous continuity between the pulmonary and aortic rings, with the infundibular septum either partially or completely missing.

Aortic valvular regurgitation appearing with a VSD occurs more frequently in cases of the subarterial infundibular type, developing in approximately 10% of cases [2]. The predisposing anatomical cause of

Practical Handbook of Echocardiography 1st edition. Edited by Jing Ping Sun, Joel Felner and John Merlino. © 2010 Blackwell Publishing Ltd.

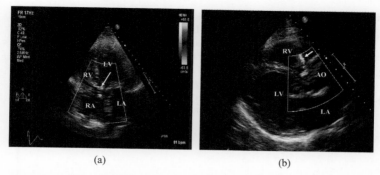

(a)   (b)

Figure 34.1. Small infundibular subarterial ventriculoseptal defect was detected by color Doppler in parasternal long-axis (a) and apical 4-chamber views (b). AO, aorta; LA, left atrium; LV, left ventricle; RA, right atrium; RV, right ventricle.

aortic prolapse is the absence of support for the anterior sigmoid, produced by the lack of the infundibular septum immediately below it. The difference in the pressure of the aorta and the pulmonary infundibula in diastole is what triggers the prolapse, and the consequent insufficiency [3]. For this reason, the risk of complications is increased with regard to the basic hemodynamic disturbance in this type of VSD.

Our case is a simple small infundibular VSD. Its location is very close to the sinus of Valsava. The treatment and progress of perforation of the sinus of Valsava are different from small VSD; the differential diagnosis between these two conditions is important.

VSDs are anatomically divided at the level of the crista supraventricularis into supracristal and infracristal defects. The subarterial infundibular type is different from the muscular infundibular type. Viewed from left side of the heart, they are positioned immediately inferior to the commissure between the right and noncoronary cusps [1].

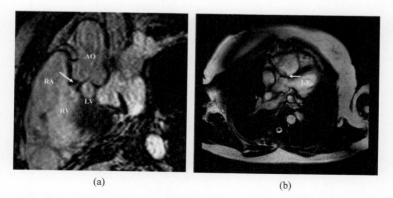

(a)   (b)

Figure 34.2. A small shunt can be seen in the magnetic resonance images (arrows point) (a and b). AO, aorta; LV, left ventricle; RA, right atrium; RV, right ventricle.

References

1. Morales GH, Antona CA, Castellanos LM, *et al.* Aortic valve complications associated with subarterial infundibular ventricular septal defect. Echocardiographic follow-up. *Rev Esp Cardiol* 2002;55:936–42.
2. Soto B, Becker AE, Moulaert AJ, Lie JT, Anderson RH. Classification of ventricular septal defects. *Br Heart J* 1980;43:332–43.
3. Tohyama K, Satomi G, Momma K. Aortic valve prolapse and aortic regurgitation associated with subpulmonic ventricular septal defect. *Am J Cardiol* 1997;79:1285–9.

35 Myocardial Bridging

Wen Xu Liu & Zhi An Li

Beijing Anzhen Hospital, Capital Medical University, Beijing, China

History

A 49-year-old male presented with a 1-year history of exercise-induced chest pain.

Physical Examination

Blood pressure was 120/80 mmHg, heart rate was 66 with regular rhythm, respiratory rate was 25, and temperature was 36.6°C. Cardiac examination revealed no murmurs with regular rhythm.

Laboratory

Chest X-ray, electrocardiography, and transthoracic echocardiography were normal. Transthoracic Doppler coronary flow imaging showed diastolic finger-tip flow pattern in the mid left anterior descending (LAD) (Figure 35.1a). The finger-tip flow profile appeared higher and sharper after sublingual use of nitroglycerin (Figure 35.1b).

Percutaneous coronary angiography showed myocardial bridging in LAD with systolic narrowing of lumen diameter with 50% of compression in systole and normal in diastole (Figure 35.2). The remaining coronary arteries were normal.

Discussion

Myocardial bridging was initially described angiographically by Portmann and Iwig [1] in 1960 and was characterized by milking effect. Intracoronary ultrasonography was applied for the diagnosis of myocardial bridging by Ge [2] in early 1990s and computed tomography in late 1990s. In recent years, transthoracic Doppler coronary flow imaging has been used for the qualitative and quantitative analysis of intracoronary hemodynamics. We initially applied color Doppler in evaluating myocardial bridging [3].

Finger-tip profile found by transthoracic coronary color Doppler is consistent with that found by intracoronary ultrasonography. This flow

Practical Handbook of Echocardiography 1st edition. Edited by Jing Ping Sun, Joel Felner and John Merlino. © 2010 Blackwell Publishing Ltd.

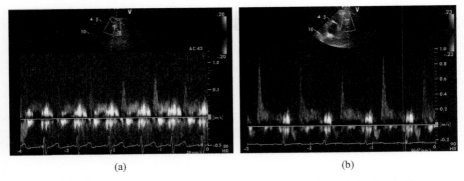

(a)   (b)

Figure 35.1. Finger-tip flow pattern at rest (a) and after sublingual use of nitroglycerin (b).

pattern is different from the pattern of normal or narrowed coronary artery, which is very specific. Ge J. found the compression of mural coronary existed until middle to late diastolic period of the cardiac cycle with intravascular ultrasonography. We consider the mechanisms of finger-tip phenomenon, combining the characteristic of coronary flow, are as follows: the resistance of coronary flow decreased as a result of the compression release in early diastole, which led to increased intracoronary flow. The ascending branch of finger-tip profile is due to antegrade coronary flow compressed by myocardium.

The finger-tip cannot be detected in some patients, and they may have finger-tip phenomenon after nitroglycerin use. As for the patients with finger-tip phenomenon at rest, the peak velocity increases, slope rate increases, and systolic retrograde flow occurs in some subjects after nitroglycerin use. Compared with other imaging techniques, transthoracic Doppler coronary flow imaging is a noninvasive, convenient, reproducible

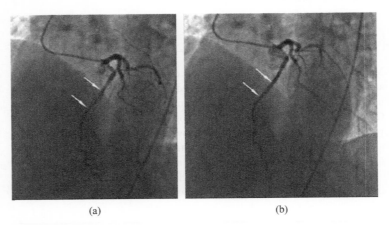

(a)   (b)

Figure 35.2. Percutaneous coronary angiography showed myocardial bridging (arrows) in left anterior descending during left ventricle systole (a) and diastole (b).

tool. Thansthoracic Doppler coronary flow imaging should be initially performed for patients with suspected coronary heart disease.

References

1. Portmann WC, Iwig J. Die intramurale koronarie im angiogramm. *Fortschr Rontgenstr* 1960;92:129–32.
2. Ge J, Jeremias A, Rupp A. New signs characteristic of myocardial bridging demonstrated by intracoronary ultrasound and Doppler. *Eur Heart J* 1999;20:1707–16.
3. Wen Xu Liu, Zhi An Li, Ya Yang *et al.* Preliminary study on myocardial bridging of the left anterior decending coronary artery by transthoracic color doppler coronary flow imaging. *Chin J Ultrasonogr* 2006;15:646–50.

36 Atrial Septal Defect

Dale Yoo & Jing Ping Sun
Emory University School of Medicine; Emory University Hospital Midtown, Atlanta, GA, USA

Studied Case

A 50-year-old female with worsening shortness of breath over a few months. Transesophageal echocardiography (TEE) study revealed a moderately dilated and moderately hypokinetic right ventricle (RV) with left-to-right flow across a 2.0 cm ventricular septal defect (Figure 36.1). She was deemed as a good candidate for percutaneous atrial septal defect (ASD) closure. The procedure was performed under TEE guidance. The defect was sized with a balloon and a 2.2-cm Amplatzer® septal occluder was secured across the ASD (Videoclip 36.1).

Discussion

ASDs are the second most commonly congenital lesions in adults (behind bicuspid aortic valves). They represent approximately 7% of all cardiac anomalies [1]. These defects are often undetected until adulthood due to the lack of prominent clinical symptoms initially. If untreated, an ASD can eventually result in RV heart failure, pulmonary hypertension, atrial arrhythmias, or paradoxical embolization and ischemic cerebral events. Often, atrial tachyarrhythmias may coexist or precede symptoms. Study has shown that the incidence of arrhythmias increase with age as well as an increase in pulmonary pressures [2]. However, it is still unclear whether atrial arrhythmias improve with the closure of the defect, although some trials have shown that atrial flutter may improve with ASD closure as opposed to atrial fibrillation, which usually remains unchanged following closure [2]. As a result, the development of an atrial tachyarrhythmia alone does not constitute an immediate need for ASD closure. Traditionally, as shown in the pediatric literature, patients with a significant pulmonary to systemic blood flow (Qp/Qs) ratio ≥ 1.5 have demonstrated the most benefit after ASD closure. One study in adults has shown that asymptomatic and mildly symptomatic patients with a Qp/Qs as low as 1.2 may also benefit from ASD closure [3].

Historically, ASDs have been closed surgically. More recently, these procedures have been accomplished with minimally invasive surgical techniques as well as a percutaneous transcatheter technique. The latter technique has been increasing in popularity due to the avoidance of cardiac

Practical Handbook of Echocardiography 1st edition. Edited by Jing Ping Sun, Joel Felner and John Merlino. © 2010 Blackwell Publishing Ltd.

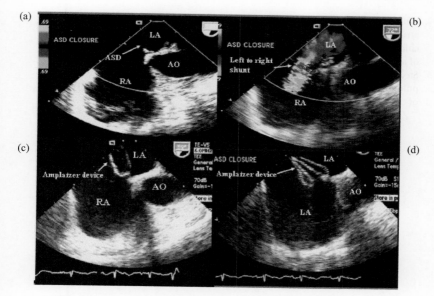

Figure 36.1. Transesophageal echocardiogram images show (a) a large atrial septal defect; (b) color Doppler image showing left to right shunt; (c) Amplatzer® device being delivered across the atrial septal defect, (d) Amplatzer® being deployed into its final position across the atrial septal defect. AO, aorta; ASD, atrial septal defect; LA, left atrium; RA, right atrium.

surgery and the associated risks. ASD repair with the transcatheter technique has been shown to have a high closure rate [4]. Unfortunately, anatomy of the defect often limits their use. Currently, transcatheter closure is limited to secundum-type defects which are less than 30 mm in size.

Patients with severe fixed pulmonary hypertension may actually do worse with ASD closure due to the need for partial right-to-left shunting of blood to decrease right-sided pressures [5]. Early diagnosis and follow-up of ASDs offers the best opportunity to avoid late complications from pulmonary hypertension, heart failure, arrhythmia, and stroke.

References

1. Rigatelli G. Congenital heart diseases in aged patients: clinical features, diagnosis, and therapeutic indications based on the analysis of a twenty five-year Medline search. *Cardiol Rev* 2005;13:293–6.
2. Berger F, Vogel M, Kramer A, *et al.* Incidence of atrial flutter/fibrillation in adults with atrial septal defect before and after surgery. *Ann Thorac Surg* 1999;68:75–8.
3. Brochu MC, Baril JF, Dore A, *et al.* Improvement in exercise capacity in asymptomatic and mildly symptomatic adults after atrial septal defect percutaneous closure. *Circulation* 2002;106:1821–6.

4. Wilson NJ, Smith J, Prommete B, *et al.* Transcatheter closure of secundum atrial septal defects with the Amplatzer septal occluder in adults and children-follow-up closure rates, degree of mitral regurgitation and evolution of arrhythmias. *Heart Lung Circ* 2008;17:318–24.
5. Steele PM, Fuster V, Cohen M, *et al.* Isolated atrial septal defect with pulmonary vascular obstructive disease–long-term follow-up and prediction of outcome after surgical correction. *Circulation* 1987;76:1037–42.

37 Ebstein's Anomaly with Wolff-Parkinson-White Syndrome

Jing Ping Sun, Xing Sheng Yang, Alicia N. Rangosch & John D. Merlino

Emory University School of Medicine; Emory University Hospital Midtown, Atlanta, GA, USA

History

A 20-year-old female was admitted because of short of breath, fatigue, and palpitations for 6 months.

Physical Examination

Blood pressure was 110/75 mmHg. Third and fourth heart sounds were heard on the precordial area, and a holosystolic murmur was heard best at the lower left parasternal area. No cyanosis or clubbing was seen.

Laboratory

Echocardiography revealed displacement of the tricuspid valve hinge point, consistent with Ebstein's anomaly, right atrium severely dilated and ventricularized, severe tricuspid regurgitation (TR) and a mid ventricular septal defect (VSD) was seen by three-dimensional view and was likely covered by tricuspid valve tissue (Figures 37.1 and 37.2, Videoclip 37.1). A small atrial septal defect (ASD) was seen in subcostal view (Videoclip 37.2). The TR velocity was 1.91 m/sec, and with an assumed right atrial pressure of 10 mmHg, the estimated pulmonary artery systolic pressure was at 24.6 mmHg. The left ventricle ejection fraction was 40%.

Eletrocardiogram demonstrated sinus rhythm, a short PR period and a delta wave suggesting pre-excitation of the Wolff-Parkinson-White-type A.

Electrophysiologic study revealed normal sinus node function and evidence of pre-excitation with a morphology suggesting a posterior right free wall pathway.

Practical Handbook of Echocardiography 1st edition. Edited by Jing Ping Sun, Joel Felner and John Merlino. © 2010 Blackwell Publishing Ltd.

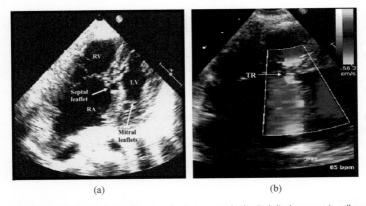

(a)   (b)

Figure 37.1. Apical 4-chamber view illustrates a marked apical displacement (small arrow) of the septal leaflet of the tricuspid valve; the distance from mitral valvular annulus is 31 mm. The tricuspid septal valve covers the ventricular septal defect can be seen (a). The tricuspid regurgitation origins from the eccentric coaptation of tricuspid valves (b). LV, left ventricle; RA, right atrium; RV, right ventricle; TR, tricuspid regurgitation.

Discussion

Ebstein's anomaly is a congenital heart disease in which the tricuspid valve is abnormally formed and it was first described by Wilhelm Ebstein in 1866. It occurs approximately 1 in 20,000 live births [1]. In Ebstein anomaly, the septal and/or posterior tricuspid valve leaflets are displaced apically into right ventricle (RV), and the anterior leaflet is elongated and may be

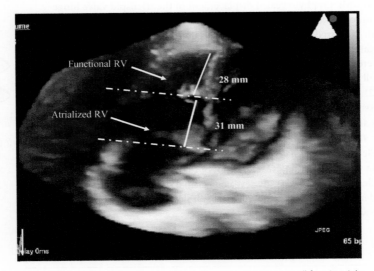

Figure 37.2. Apical 4-chamber view (three-dimensional) shows a small function right ventricle; the ratio of atrialized and functional right ventricle is 1:1. RV, right ventricle.

adherent to the wall of the chamber. This leads to atrialization of RV with a variable degree of malformation and displacement of the anterior leaflet.

Ebstein anomaly is commonly associated with other congenital structural, or conduction system disease, including ASD or patent foramen oval, valvular lesions, and accessory conduction pathways. All of these abnormalities are seen in our case; there is a VSD which appears to be closed by the septal leaflet of the tricuspid valve.

Echocardiography is the most useful tool in detecting Ebstein's anomaly. Apical displacement of the septal leaflet in apical 4-chamber (A4-ch) view has been shown as the single most diagnostic feature of this anomaly [2]. Normally, in the A4-ch view, the septal leaflet of the tricuspid inserts into interventricular septum slightly (<1 cm) lower than the septal insertion of the anterior mitral leaflet. A displacement index of ≥ 8 mm/m^2 appeared to more clearly separate patients with Ebstein's anomaly from another forms of RV volume overload [3]. Morphologic characteristics associated with lower function classification include (1) a small functional RV (atrialized/functional RV ratio of >0.5); (2) extreme septal leaflet displacement; (3) absent septal leaflet; (4) displacement anterior tricuspid leaflet; (5) tethering of the anterior leaflet; and (6) aneurismal dilation of the right ventricular outflow tract. Moderate or severe TR is also associated with a lower function classification [4].

Surgical repair of Ebstein's anomaly can improve functional class and exercise tolerance, and reduces the incidence of supraventricular tachyarrhythmias [5].

References

1. Patanè S, Marte F, Di Bella G, *et al.* Ebstein's anomaly in adult. *Int J Cardiol* 2009 Jul 24;136(1):e6–7.
2. Ports TA, Silverman NH, Schiller NB. Two dimensional echocardiographic assessment of Ebstein's anomaly. *Circulation* 1978;58:336–43.
3. Stulak JM, Deaani JA, Danie GK. Surgical management of Ebstein's anomaly. *Semin Thorac Cardiovas Surg Pediatr Card Surg Annu,* 2007:105–11.
4. Weyman AE. *Principle and Practice of Echocardiography,* 2nd edition. Philadelphia: Lea & Febiger, 1994. p. 842.
5. Filsoufi F, Salzberg SP, Abascal V, *et al..* Surgical management of functional tricuspid regurgitation with a new remodeling annuloplasty ring. *Mt Sinai J Med* 2006;73:874–9.

38 Double-Chambered Right Ventricle Associated with Ventricular Septal Defect

Jing Ping Sun & John D. Merlino

Emory University School of Medicine; Emory University Hospital Midtown, Atlanta, GA, USA

History

A 46-year-old gentleman has a history of cardiac surgery for ventricular septal defect (VSD) as a youth and had a right parietal cortical stroke in 1996.

Physical Examination

Heart rate was 76/minute; blood pressure was 140/85 mmHg. Cardiac rhythm was regular and there was a harsh intense ejection murmur in the low external border.

Laboratory

Transthoracic echocardiography: Apical 4-chamber view indicates a prominent hypertrophied muscle band divide the right ventricle (RV) cavity into a proximal and a distal chamber and dilated right atrium (Figure 38.1a, Videoclip 38.1a). Transesophageal echocardiography (TEE) in the longitudinal plane illustrates the turbulent flow signals consistent with obstruction are produced by hypertrophied muscle bundle running transversely through the RV body (Figure 38.1b, Videoclip 38.1b). Pulse wave Doppler recording with the sample volume in the orifice of hypertrophied muscle band and the systolic and diastolic signals are well seen. The peak early diastolic velocity is 156 cm/sec and gradient between two RV chambers is 10 mmHg estimated by continues wave Doppler (Figure 38.2). A hypertrophied muscle bundle divide the RV cavity into two chambers. The muscle bundle run between an area located in the ventricular septum, beneath the level of the septal leaflet of the tricuspid valve, and the anterior wall of the RV demonstrated by TEE in the longitudinal plane; a right to left shunt through the patent foramen ovale (PFO) is indicated by TEE with color Doppler (Figure 38.3). The diagnosis,

Practical Handbook of Echocardiography 1st edition. Edited by Jing Ping Sun, Joel Felner and John Merlino. © 2010 Blackwell Publishing Ltd.

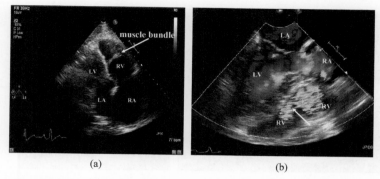

(a)   (b)

Figure 38.1. Transthoracic echocardiography: Apical 4-chamber view indicates a prominent hypertrophied muscle band (arrow) divide the right ventricular cavity into a proximal and a distal chamber; the right atrium is dilated (a). Transesophageal echocardiography in the longitudinal plane illustrated the turbulent flow signals (arrow) consistent with obstruction are produced by hypertrophied muscle bundle running transversely through the right ventricle body (b). LA, left atrium; LV, left ventricle; RA, right atrium; RV, right ventricle.

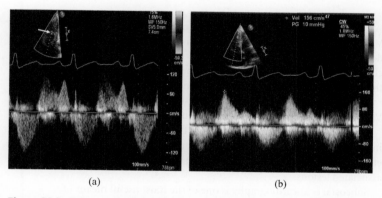

(a)   (b)

Figure 38.2. Pulse wave Doppler recording with the sample volume in the orifice of hypertrophied muscle band (arrow), the systolic and diastolic signals are well seen (a). The peak early diastolic velocity is 156 cm/sec and estimated gradient between two right ventricle chambers is 10 mmHg (b).

as summarized in the findings of echocardiography, is double-chambered right ventricle (DCRV) associated with VSD (repaired) and PFO.

Discussion

DCRV is a cardiac anomaly in which an anomalous muscle bundles divide the RV into a high-pressure proximal chamber and a lower-pressure distal chamber.

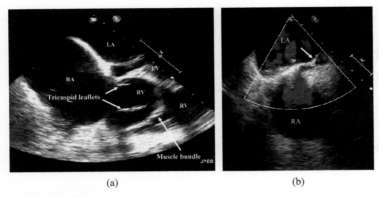

(a)   (b)

Figure 38.3. A hypertrophied muscle bundle divide the right ventricle cavity into a proximal and a distal chamber. The muscle bundle (arrow) run between an area located in the ventricular septum, beneath the level of the septal leaflet of the tricuspid valve, and the anterior wall of the right ventricle demonstrated by transesophageal echocardiography in the longitudinal plane (a). A right to left shunt (arrow) through the patent foramen oval is indicated by transesophageal echocardiography with color Doppler (b). LA, left atrium; LV, left ventricle; RA, right atrium; RV, right ventricle.

Associated defects are present in approximately 80–90% of patients; a VSD involves the membranous septum is the most common defect described. A VSD may communicate with either the proximal or the distal chamber, leading to a greater shunt in the latter situation [1,2]. In our case, the VSD communicated with the proximal chamber.

The next most common associated lesion is pulmonary valve stenosis. Various other associations have also been reported.

Echocardiography is a useful tool for the complete diagnosis. It is important, when evaluating the patient, cardiologists should make an effort to image the entire RV; they also have to be aware of the possible associated lesions.

Subcostal echocardiography is one of the most useful means of visualizing right ventricular outflow tract and can facilitate adequate visualization of RV.

When DCRV is diagnosed in the adult patient, McElhinney *et al.* recommend repair in almost all cases having DCRV with symptoms or associated lesions, or asymptomatic patients with obstruction of a significant degree (>40 mmHg gradient) [3]. Long-term follow-up studies have shown that patients do well after repair of DCRV, although cases with recurrent obstruction have been described [4].

References

1. Pongiglione G, Freedom RM, Cook D, Rowe RD. Mechanism of acquired right ventricular outflow tract obstruction in patients with ventricular septal defect. *Am J Cardiol* 1982;50:776–80.
2. Forster JW, Humphries JO. Right ventricular anomalous muscle bundles. *Circulation* 1971;43:115–27.

3. McElhinney DB, Chatterjee KM, Reddy VM. Double-chambered right ventricle presenting in adulthood. *Ann Thorac Surg* 2000;70:124–7.
4. Moran AM, Hornberger LK, Jonas RA, Keane JF. Development of double-chambered right ventricle after repair of tetralogy of Fallot. *J Am Coll Cardiol* 1998;31:1127–33.

39 Unroofed Coronary Sinus Defect

Jing Ping Sun[1], Xing Sheng Yang[1], Joel M. Felner[2], Robert D. O'Donnell Jr.[1] & John D. Merlino[1]

[1] Emory University School of Medicine; Emory University Hospital Midtown, Atlanta, GA, USA
[2] Grady Memorial Hospital; Emory University School of Medicine, Atlanta, GA, USA

History

A 40-year-old female presented with diffuse body pains and chills.

Physical Examination

Blood pressure was 110/70 mmHg. Heart rate was 98 beats/min with a regulate rhythm.

Cardiac examination was unremarkable.

Laboratory Study

Echocardiogram: The significantly dilated coronary sinus with high velocity flow into right atrium (RA) was noted in parasternal right ventricle (RV) inflow tract view (Figure 39.1a). Apical 4-chamber view shows high velocity flow from entrance of unroofed coronary sinus (URCS) run into RA with upper direction (Figure 39.1b). Pulse wave Doppler recording showed the velocity of coronary sinus entrance flow was almost 1.2 m/sec (Figure 39.2).

Doppler recordings of left and right ventricular outflow tract; Qp/Qs = 1.9 indicated there was a left to right shunt (Figure 39.3).

Figure 39.4 illustrates (a) diagram of unroofed coronary sinus defect (UCSD). (b) Three-dimensional (3D) apical short-axis view (crop from basal) shows the relation among the coronary sinus, defect of sinus (white arrow) and left atrium (LA). The RV and atrial cavity size was mildly enlarged.

Videoclip 39.1 shows coronary sinus flow from 3D apical set with color Doppler crop from post.

Practical Handbook of Echocardiography 1st edition. Edited by Jing Ping Sun, Joel Felner and John Merlino. © 2010 Blackwell Publishing Ltd.

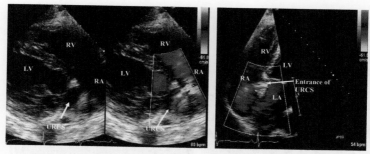

Figure 39.1. Parasternal right ventricular inflow tract view shows the significantly dilated coronary sinus (arrow) with a high-velocity flow (arrow) into right atrium (left). Apical 4-chamber view shows high velocity flow from entrance of unroofed coronary sinus run into right atrium with upper direction (right).LA, left atrium; LV, left ventricle; RA, right atrium; RV, right ventricle; URCS, unroofed coronary sinus.

MRI image demonstrates the blood flow enter the RA from coronary sinus entrance with lower velocity during atrial systole and high velocity during atrial diastole (Videoclip 39.2).

Cardiac catheterization demonstrated no obstructive coronary disease; right cardiac catheterization indicated an oxygen saturation of 68% in the

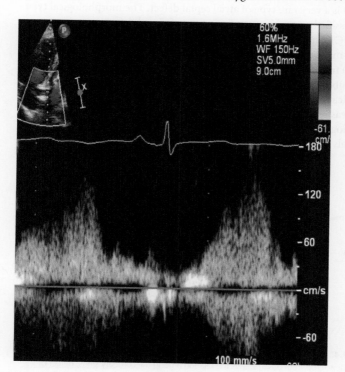

Figure 39.2. Pulse wave Doppler recording shows the velocity of coronary sinus entrance flow was almost 1.2 m/sec.

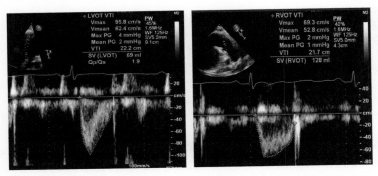

Figure 39.3. Doppler recordings of left and right ventricular outflow tract; Qp/Qs = 1.9 indicates there is a left to right shunt.

right atrium, the oxygen saturation increased to 75% at the mid right atrium. The shunt fraction was found to be 1.45:1.

Discussion

An UCSD is a very rare type of atrial septal defect. The morphological type can be classified as: type I, completely unroofed with left superior vena cava (LSVC); type II, completely unroofed without LSVC; type III, partial unroofed mid portion; and type IV, partial unroofed terminal portion [1].

The 3D transthoracic echocardiography (TTE) acquired from the apical four-chamber view were cropped using multiple planes and angulations. A communication between the LA and a prominent coronary sinus (CS) could be easily identified on transverse cropping of the 3D echocardiogram. Three-dimensional color Doppler flow imaging showed flow signals moving from the LA into the CS and then into the RA. Thus, a

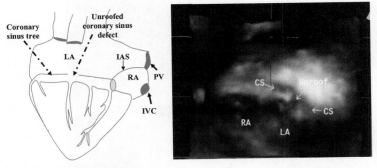

Figure 39.4. Diagram of a unroofed coronary sinus defect. Three-dimensional apical short-axis view (crop from basal) shows the relation among the coronary sinus, defect of sinus (white arrow) and left atrium. CS, coronary sinus; IAS, interatrial septum; IVC, inferior vena cava; LA, left atrium; PV, pulmonic valve; RA, right atrium.

definitive diagnosis of UCSD could be made using 3D TTE. This was because both the B-mode and color Doppler 3D TTE could be cropped and viewed in various planes and angulations [2].

In our case, a dilated coronary sinus vein with high-velocity flow entrance into RA with upper direction and a communication between the LA and a prominent CS was identified by two-dimensional and 3D TTE. magnetic resonance image indicated the blood flow enter RA with lower velocity during atrial systole and high velocity during atrial diastole, which supports the flow is from the coronary sinus. Right side catheterization also found there was a left to right shunt. All of these results suggested the diagnose is type III UCSD.

References

1. Ootaki Y, Yamaguchi M, Yoshimura N, *et al.* Unroofed coronary sinus syndrome: diagnosis, classification, and surgical treatment. *J Thorac Cardiovasc Surg* 2003;126:1655–6.
2. Singh A., Nanda NC, Romp RL, *et al.* Assessment of surgically unroofed coronary sinus by live/real time three-dimensional transthoracic echocardiography. *Echocardiography* 2007;24:74–76.

40 Membranous Ventricular Septal Defect with Bicuspid Aortic Valve

Jing Ping Sun, Xing Sheng Yang & John D. Merlino
Emory University School of Medicine; Emory University Hospital Midtown, Atlanta, GA, USA

History

A 37-year-old male with a known ventricular septal defect (VSD) and a bicuspid aortic valve with mild aortic regurgitation (AR) referred for elective repair of VSD. The patient reported a patent ductus arteriosus (PDA) closured in infancy.

Physical Examination

A 3/6 holosystolic murmur was present along the left sternal border with wide radiation throughout the precordium. Lungs were clear to auscultation and percussion.

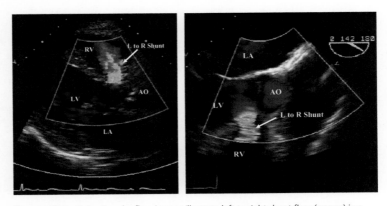

Figure 40.1. Color Doppler flow images illustrate left to right shunt flow (arrows) in a patient with membranous ventricular septal defect. RV, right ventricle; LV, left ventricle; AO, aorta; LA, left atrium.

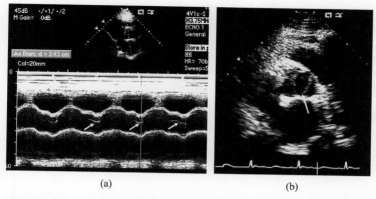

(a)   (b)

Figure 40.2. M-mode echocardiographic images illustrate the eccentric closing line (arrows) of aortic valve (a). Aortic valvular short-axis view indicates the opening of bicuspid valve; it is like a fish's mouth (b, arrow) in the same patient with membranous ventricular septal defect.

Laboratory

Echocardiography: The left ventricle is mildly dilated. There is a perimembranous VSD present with left to right flow (Figure 40.1, Videoclip 40.1). The VSD measures about 1.1 cm with left to right shunt. The overall left ventricular function is normal. The aortic valve is functionally bicuspid with the right and noncoronary cusps appearing fused (Figure 40.2). The aortic valve leaflets are thickened with mild to moderate AR (Videoclip 40.2). The right ventricle size and function are normal. There is a mild to moderate amount of tricuspid regurgitation. The left atrium is enlarged.

He underwent an elective closure of membranous VSD without complications.

Discussion

Ventricular septal defects are classified according to the location of the defect in one of the four ventricular components: the inlet septum, trabecular septum, outlet/infundibular septum, or membranous septum [1]. VSD is the most common congenital heart defect in the first three decades of life, with an incidence of 1.5–3.5 cases for every 1000 infants. Membranous VSD is the most common type, accounting for as many as 50% of VSD cases identified in most surgical or autopsy series. Perimembranous VSDs may spontaneously decrease in size and eventually close. Closure rates as high as 50% have been reported in some series [2].

Some studies have identified an increased incidence of bicuspid aortic valve in patients with VSD because endocardial cushion remodeling contributes to the formation of both semilunar valves and ventricular septation.

The combination of VSD with PDA is not very uncommon. Accurate estimation of the frequency of occurrence cannot be made recently.

The present case has PDA, bicuspid aortic valve and VSD; one patient may have more than one or two congenital defects. A thorough echocardiographic study is always important to detect the possible abnormalities.

References

1. Taylor MD, Eidem BW. Ventricular septal defect, perimembranous. *Mayo Clin Proc* 2007;82:65–7.
2. Hoffman JI, Rudolph AM. The natural history of ventricular septal defects in infancy. *Am J Cardiol* 1965;16(5):634–53

41 Atrial Septal Aneurysm

Shawn X. Yang

Memorial Hermann Southwest Medical Center, Houston, TX, USA

History

A 60-year-old man was having weakness in his left leg, which had progressed to the point where he was unable to stand with suspicion of cardiogenic embolism.

Physical Examination

Blood pressure was 100/64 mmHg. The strength in his left lower limb was decreased.

Echocardiography

Transthoracic echocardiography (TTE) revealed that left and right atria and ventricles are normal in size and function. An atrial septal aneurysm

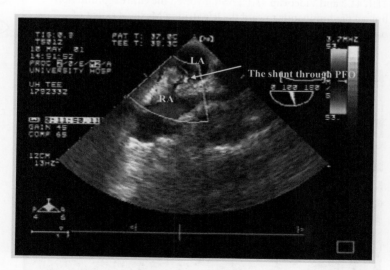

Figure 41.1. Original transesophageal echocardiography demonstrating an atrial septal aneurysm and a shunt through patent foramen ovale. LA, left atrium; RA, right atrium.

Practical Handbook of Echocardiography 1st edition. Edited by Jing Ping Sun, Joel Felner and John Merlino. © 2010 Blackwell Publishing Ltd.

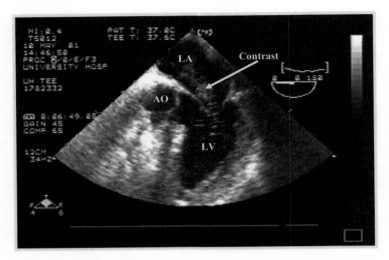

Figure 41.2. Transesophageal echocardiogram image shows the contrast through patent foramen ovale into the left atrium and left ventricle. AO, aorta; LA, left atrium; LV, left ventricle.

(ASA) was noted in the apical 4 chamber and subcustal views. For more information, the patient underwent transesophageal echocardiography (TEE). Contrast TEE and color Doppler revealed an ASA associated with a right-to-left shunt through patent foramen oval in the aneurysm (Figure 41.1, 41.2 and Videoclip 41.1); ASA involved the entire septum. ASA bulged predominantly toward the left atrium. Maximal extent of oscillation was 17 mm (Figure 41.3 and Videoclip 41.2).

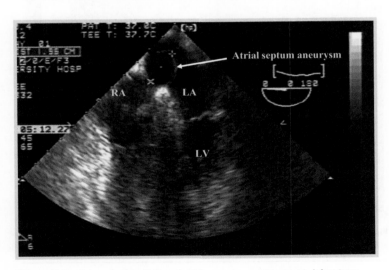

Figure 41.3. The maximal oscillation of atrial aneurysm was 17 mm. LA, left atrium; LV, left ventricle; RA, right atrium.

Discussion

ASA is a localized deformity of the interatrial septum, generally at the level of the fossa ovale, which bulges into the right or left atrium or both. ASA was initially thought to be a rare congenital abnormality; however, with the advent of two-dimensional echocardiography and more recently, with the widespread use of TEE it is more easily and more frequently identified in patients.

The prevalence of ASA varies; TTE studies estimate the rate to be between 0.12 and 0.54% [1]. In a large autopsy series the prevalence reported was 1%. Studies using TEE have demonstrated a prevalence between 3 and 8% [2,3].

ASA has been associated with congenital heart diseases such as patent foramen ovale (PFO), atrial septal defects, ventricular septal defects, valvular prolapse, PFO, Ebstein's anomaly, and tricuspid and pulmonary atresia as well as acquired heart diseases including valvular disease, cardiomyopathy, systemic and pulmonary hypertension, ischemic heart disease, arrhythmias, and thrombus formation. More recently a number of studies found an association between ASA and cerebrovascular events of embolic origin, including transient ischemic attacks and cerebrovascular accidents.

Diagnostic Criteria for ASA

The cutoff point between a slightly redundant atrial septum and an ASA is somewhat arbitrary. A cutoff criteria reported in an autopsy study by Silver and Dorsey [5], a protrusion of the aneurysm > 10 mm beyond the plane of the atrial septum into either the right or the left atrium. The criteria of an ASA diagnosed by echocardiography include a 15-mm diameter at the base of aneurysm and excursion of 11 mm into either atrial chamber from the plane of the atrial septum obtained from parasternal, apical, subcostal, or transesophageal transducer position [3]. Sixteen aneurysms of the septum primum were found at autopsy among 1,578 adults. Most occurred in individuals in their fifth or sixth decade [4].

ASA was found and defined as a possible source of embolism in 173 of 2037 patients (8.4%) with previous ischemic stroke and/or peripheral arterial embolism [5].

Our case had a simple ASA and PFO without another abnormality, but his mild stroke may be related to the right to left shunt.

References

1. Longhini C, Brunazzi MC, Musacci G, *et al.* Atrial septal aneurysm: echopolycardiographic study. *Am J Cardiol* 1985 October;56(10):653–6.
2. Schneider B, Hanrath P, Vogel P, *et al.* Improved morphologic characterization of atrial septal aneurysm by transesophageal echocardiography: relation to cerebrovascular events. *J Am Coll Cardiol* 1990 October;16(4):1000–1009.

3. Pearson AC, Nagelhout D, Castello R, *et al.* Atrial septal aneurysm and stroke: a transesophageal echocardiographic study. *J Am Coll Cardiol* 1991 November;18(5):1223–9.

4. Silver MD, Dorsey JS. Aneurysms of the septum primum in adults. *Arch Pathol Lab Med* 1978;102:62–5.

5. Mirode A, Tribouilloy C, Boey S, *et al.* Aneurysmes du septum interauriculaire: apport de l'echographie transoesophagienne: relation avec les accidents systèmique emboliques. *Ann Cardiol Angeiol (Paris)* 1993;42:7–12.

42 Interventricular Membranous Septal Aneurysm

Jing Ping Sun, Xing Sheng Yang & John D. Merlino
Emory University School of Medicine; Emory University Hospital Midtown, Atlanta, GA, USA

History

A 20-year-old female was admitted due to new onset shortness of breath and chest pain.

Physical Examination

Blood pressure was 120/82 mmHg. Heart rate was 72 beats/min. A grade 2/6 holosystolic murmur was audible, which radiated to the left axilla.

Laboratory

Transthoracic echocardiography: The LV (left ventricle) is normal in size and shape; there is a 1-cm diameter aneurysm of the membranous interventricular septum (AMIS) (Figure 42.1, Videoclip 42.1). An entire AMIS is seen in the apical long-axis view with color Doppler (Videoclip 42.2). These two videoclips indicate that this aneurysm is entirely without defect. The LV ejection fraction is estimated at 55–60%. The right ventricle (RV) size and function are normal. The left and right atriums are normal in size.

Discussion

Aneurysms of the membranous of interventricular septum are relatively rare lesions and are probably of congenital origin as is in the current case. There is now evidence to suggest that aneurysms may develop in the course of spontaneous partial or complete closure of ventricular septal defects (VSDs), although their exact anatomic basis is controversial [1]. Some studies have reported that aneurysm formation is associated with diminution in the functional size of membranous VSDs, and considered that the formation of aneurysms of the membranous septum is one mechanism of closure of VSD [2].

Practical Handbook of Echocardiography 1st edition. Edited by Jing Ping Sun,
Joel Felner and John Merlino. © 2010 Blackwell Publishing Ltd.

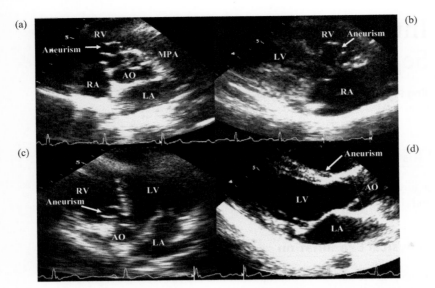

Figure 42.1. There is a 1-cm diameter aneurysm of the membranous interventricular septum, which is well seen in the parasternal short-axis view (a), right ventricle inflow view (b), apical 5-chamber view (c) and parasternal long-axis view (d). RV, right ventricle; RA, right atrium; AO, aorta; LA, left atrium; LV, Left ventricle; MPA, main pulmonary artery.

Most often there has been a small left-to-right shunt through perforations in the aneurysm and auscultation indicates a VSD. Ventricular septal aneurysms which are not perforated, such as our case, may cause no murmur at all or be associated with a nonspecific murmur generated within the aneurysm itself, by protrusion of the aneurysm into the right ventricular outflow tract (RVOT). Clinically, aneurysms may have the potential to reduce ventricular size, and they are further complicated by rupture of the aneurysm and by promoting tricuspid regurgitation, ventricular outflow tract obstruction, aortic valve prolapse, and bacterial endocarditis.

Echocardiography can be an accurate noninvasive method of detecting ventricular septal aneurysms. These echoes seem to be originating from the base (membranous) of the septum in systole and protruded in RVOT.

For maximum diagnostic accuracy, multiple two-dimensional echocardiographic views must be used. The thinness and rapid motion of the septal aneurysms and overall cardiac motion may cause a single view to miss the aneurysm. The long-axis and apical 4-chamber views are able to be the most helpful in visualizing the area of the membranous septum. Careful cranial transducer angulation from the long-axis and apical views will allow the best identification of the membranous septum. The location of the aneurysm and the dynamic nature of its bulging into RV during systole can be appreciated with this technique.

References

1. Miora KP, Hildner FJ, Cohen LS, *et al.* Aneurysm of the membranous ventricular septum. A mechanism for spontaneous closure of ventricular septal defect. *N Eng J Med* 1970;283:58–62.
2. Lambert ME, Widlansky S, Frankin EA, *et al.* Natural history of ventricular septal defects associated with ventricular septal aneurysms. *Am Heart J* 1974;88:566–72.

43 Congenital Interrupted Aortic Arch

Jian Hua Wang & Gui Chun Ding
The Second Military Medical University, Shanghai; The General Hospital of Beijing Military Command of PLA, Beijing, China

Case History

A 4-year-old girl with heart murmurs for 3 years presented for further diagnosis.

Physical Examination

Blood pressure was 96/60 mmHg, heart rate was 125 bpm with regular rhythm, respiratory rate was 20 and temperature was 36.9°C. On cardiac examination, there were heart murmurs of 3/6 degree at left side of the chest.

Laboratory

The electrocardiogram indicated the hypertrophy of right atrium (RA) and right ventricle (RV). Chest X-ray revealed the enlargement of the RA and RV with possible infection of the left lung.

Transthoracic echocardiography (TTE) findings included (1) suprasternal notch long-axis view of aortic arch with color Doppler illustrating the interrupted aortic arch (IAA) and descending aorta (Figure 43.1); (2) parasternal short-axis view with color Doppler found the patent duct artery (PDA) between descending aorta and left pulmonary artery (Figure 43.2); (3) apical 4-chamber view showing the stenosis of the mitral valves caused by valvular deformation; continuous wave Doppler recordings of mitral valvular jet velocity from A4-ch view, the peak velocity was 2.27 m/sec and the maximal gradient was 20.6 mmHg (Figure 43.3).

The diagnosis of IAA in this patient was confirmed by three-dimensional computed tomography angiography and aortic angiography.

Management: Because of the high risk of operation, the parents of the patient refused to give consent to operation.

Practical Handbook of Echocardiography 1st edition. Edited by Jing Ping Sun, Joel Felner and John Merlino. © 2010 Blackwell Publishing Ltd.

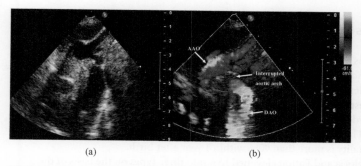

Figure 43.1. Suprasternal notch long-axis view of aortic arch (a), and with color Doppler (b) illustrating the interrupted aortic arch and descending arota. AAO, ascending aorta; DAO, descending aorta.

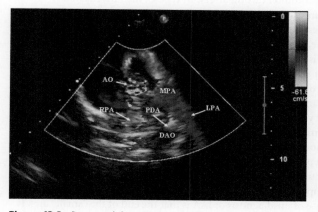

Figure 43.2. Parasternal short-axis view with color Doppler illustrating patent duct artery between descending aorta and left pulmonary artery. AO, aorta; DAO, descending aorta; LPA, left pulmonary artery; MPA, main pulmonary artery; PDA, patent duct artery; RPA, right pulmonary artery.

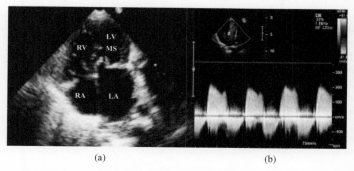

Figure 43.3. Apical 4-chamber view shows the stenosis of the mitral valves caused by valvular deformation (a). Continuous wave Doppler recordings of mitral valvular jet velocity from the apical 4-chamber view. The peak velocity was 2.27 m/sec and the maximal gradient was 20.6 mmHg (b). LA, left atrium; LV, left ventricle; MS, mitral valve stenosis; RA, right atrium; RV, right ventricle.

Discussion

IAA is a malformation of aortic arch with disconnection between ascending aorta and descending aorta. IAA is a rare disease with an incidence of 0.02–0.003‰ and it is less than 1.3% of all congenital heart disease [1]. The majority of IAA are complicated with other cardiovascular disorders such as ventricular septal defect (VSD), patent ductus arteriosus, etc. The prognosis of IAA is fatal, and without proper treatment, the mortality is more than 90% within 1 year after birth.

Celoria and Patton classified IAA into three types on the basis of the location of interruption: in type A, the interruption is distal to the origin of subclavian artery. In type B, the interruption is between left subclavian artery and left common carotid artery. In type C, the interruption is between innominate artery and left common carotid artery. PDA is commonly presented to supply blood to descending aorta, and in a rare case of absence, the blood supply of descending aorta depends on collateral arteries. VSD is often complicated with IAA, especially in type B. Other cardiovascular malformation complicated with IAA included the transposition of the great arteries, single ventricle, trunks artery, atriaventricular septal defect, hypoplastic left heart syndrome, double-outlet ventricle, etc. [2].

TTE is the main modality for the diagnosis of IAA and can provide enough diagnostic information in most cases as long as the image quality is acceptable. In patient with VSD and severe pulmonary hypertension, the left to right shunt at ventricular level is a clue to IAA. The supersternal view is the most important one to detect the aortic arch and its branch arteries. The main cause of misdiagnosis of IAA is that the end of the "small" arch is not viewed clearly while dilated pulmonary-PDA-descending aorta looks like the descending part of the aortic arch.

Computed tomography angiography and aortic angiography can provide definite diagnosis for IAA.

References

1. Morriss MJH, McNamara DG. Coarctation of aorta and interrupted aortic arch. In: Garson Jr. A, Bricker JT, Fisher DJ, *et al.* (eds) *The Science and Pratice of Pediatric Cardiology*, 2nd edition. Baltimore: William & Wilkins, 1998, pp. 1317–46.
2. Yan Ling Liu, Jian Ran Xiong. *Clinical Echocardiography*, 2nd edition. Beijing: Science Press, 2007, pp. 539–49.

44 Aortopulmonary Window and Atrioventricular Septal Defect

Leilei Cheng[1], Xianhong Shu[1] & Jing Ping Sun[2]

[1] Shanghai Cardiovascular Diseases Institute, Zhongshan Hospital, Fudan University, Shanghai, China

[2] Emory University School of Medicine; Emory University Hospital Midtown, Atlanta, GA, USA

History

A 14-year-old boy presented with shortness of breath and a history of congenital heart disease since he was born.

Physical Examination

The patient appeared to have malnutrition and delayed development. Blood pressure was 110/80 mmHg, heart rate was 85 bmp with regular rhythm, respiratory rate was 25 and temperature was 36.8°C. His heart had grade 3 continuous machinery murmurs in aortic area.

Laboratory

The chest X-ray revealed a large heart shadow. Computed tomography demonstrated the patient had enlarged heart, one large defect between aorta and main pulmonary artery, a very big ventricular septal defect (VSD), and a bicuspid aortic valve.

Transthoracic echocardiography: Aortopulmonary window could be well seen between the ascending aorta and the main pulmonary artery from parasternal short-axis (PSA) view (Figure 44.1, Videoclip 44.1), and from the suprasternal fossa view (Figure 44.2a). A perimembrane VSD with left to right shunt was noted from apical 4-chamber view (Figure 44.3, Videoclip 44.2). The bicuspid aortic valve with normal function was confirmed from the PSA view. The pulmonary pressure estimated by continuous wave Doppler of tricuspid regurgitation was 110 mmHg.

Color Doppler echocardiography showed the blood flow from ascending aorta to main pulmonary artery. It was continuous shunt during systole and diastole. Because aortopulmonary (AP) window was large, the velocity of the shunt was not high and presented as laminar flow.

Practical Handbook of Echocardiography 1st edition. Edited by Jing Ping Sun, Joel Felner and John Merlino. © 2010 Blackwell Publishing Ltd.

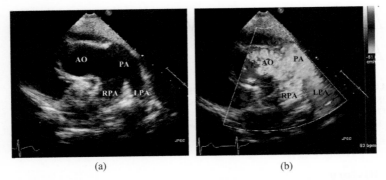

(a) (b)

Figure 44.1. Aortopulmonary window can be well seen between the ascending aorta and the main pulmonary artery from the parasternal short-axis view (a). Color Doppler echocardiography shows the shunt from ascending aorta into main pulmonary artery (b). AO, aorta; LPA, left pulmonary artery; PA, pulmonary artery; RPA, right pulmonary artery.

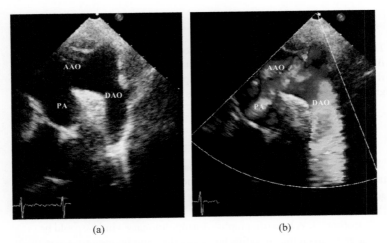

(a) (b)

Figure 44.2. Aortopulmonary window (28 mm) can be well seen between the ascending aorta and the main pulmonary artery from the suprasternal fossa view (a). Color Doppler echocardiography shows the shunt from ascending aorta into pulmonary artery (b). AAO, ascending aorta; DAO, descending aorta; PA, pulmonary artery.

Management

The patient underwent a successful chest operation without complications.

Discussion

AP window is a communication between the ascending aorta and the main pulmonary artery, in the presence of two separate arterial valves arising

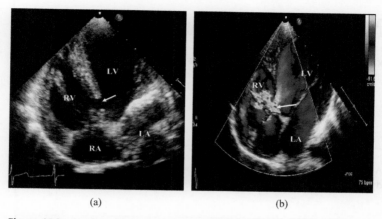

(a)   (b)

Figure 44.3. A perimembrane ventricular septal defect (arrow) detected from apical 4-chamber view (a). There was left-to-right shunt (arrow) through perimembrane ventricular septal defect during early systole (b). LA, left atrium; LV, left ventricle; RA, right atrium; RV, right ventricle.

from separate subarterial ventricular outflow tracts. It is a rare anomaly that accounts for approximately 0.1–0.2% of all congenital heart diseases [1].

The embryogenesis of AP window is related to incomplete fusion or malalignment of the right and left conotruncal ridges, which normally completely septate the truncus arteriosus between the fifth and eighth weeks of intrauterine life. This AP window with various arterial abnormalities, including transposition of the great arteries and aortic interruption, anomalous origin of a coronary artery, VSD, atrial septal defect, patent ductus arteriosus, pulmonary or aortic atresia, etc.

Aortopulmonary septal defect's clinical presentation is dependent on the size of the defect and the associated lesions. It can be confused with other defects. Soares *et al.* reported that the group of 18 patients had aortopulmonary septal defect. Diagnosis was established by echocardiography in 11 patients (61.2%) [2]. The diagnosis of aortopulmonary septal defect could be masked by other important associated defects [3]. A complete echocardiogram should be performed carefully to avoid missing any associated abnormalities. The AP window was associated with the perimembrane VSD, and bicuspid aortic valve in our case.

The operation should be performed as soon as the AP window confirmed to prevent the irreversible arterial pulmonary hypertension.

References

1. Kutsche LM, Van Mierop LH. Anatomy and pathogenesis of aorticopulmonary septal defect. *Am J Cardiol* 1987;59(5):443–7.
2. Soares AM, Atik E, Cortêz TM, *et al.* Aortopulmonary window. Clinical and surgical assessment of 18 cases. *Arq Bras Cardiol* 1999;73(1):59–74.
3. Bertolini A, Dalmonte P, Bava GL. Aortopulmonary septal defects. A review of the literature and report of ten cases. *J Cardiovasc Surg* 1994;35(3):207–13.

45 Marfan's Syndrome

Xing Sheng Yang[1], Jing Ping Sun[1] & Joel M. Felner[2]

[1] Emory University School of Medicine; Emory University Hospital Midtown, Atlanta, GA, USA
[2] Grady Memorial Hospital; Emory University School of Medicine, Atlanta, GA, USA

History

A 30-year-old man was admitted because of chest pain and exertional dyspnea.

Physical Examination

Patient was tall with long and thin fingers. Blood pressure was 120/65 mmHg; heart rate was 82/minute. Apex impulse was in normal location with presystolic and sustained systolic motion. Auscultation showed S2 normally split; 3/6 late-systolic murmur with prominent mid-systolic clicks in the apex area. Peripheral pulses were normal bilaterally.

Laboratory

Chest X-ray essentially unchanged. Electrocardiogram revealed frequent unifocal ventricular premature beats. Transesophageal echocardiography documented a marked enlargement of the aortic-root diameter and the aortic wall appeared thin with aortic regurgitation (AR) and dissection (Figure 45.1, Videoclip 45.1), as well as left ventricle (LV) and left atrium enlargement with a normal ejection fraction.

Discussion

Marfan's syndrome is a generalized disorder of connective tissue inherited as an autosomal dominant trait with a high degree of penetrance. It occurs at equal rates in both sexes, and there is no racial preponderance. The prevalence of Marfan's syndrome is 4–6 per hundred thousand subjects [1].

Aortic dilatation due to the weakening of the aorta media can start as early as the first year of life. However, it may be delayed until the fifth decade of life, and usually occurs first in the coronary sinus [2]. The involvement of the cardiovascular system (mitral valve prolapse, AR, aorta root dilatation, and dissection) accounts for 90% of deaths attributed to Marfan's syndrome.

Practical Handbook of Echocardiography 1st edition. Edited by Jing Ping Sun,
Joel Felner and John Merlino. © 2010 Blackwell Publishing Ltd.

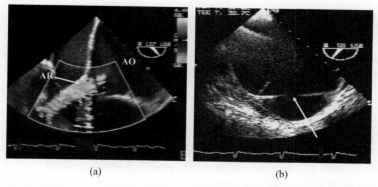

(a)   (b)

Figure 45.1. Transesophageal echocardiography long-axis view shows the dilated aortic root with aortic regurgitation (a), and short-axis view illustrates the dilated aortic root with dissection (b, arrow). AO, aorta; AR, aortic regurgitation.

Fetal echocardiography has typical features especially in those with family history of Marfan's syndrome. Regurgitation of atrioventricular valve and dilatation of aortic root are findings that are suggestive of the condition [1].

The characteristics of echocardiogram include (1) the aortic root is typically dilated and the aortic walls appear thin; (2) the pattern of aortic root dilation is unique in that it involves the annulus, sinuses of Valsalva; (3) the aortic leaflets are elongated and may prolapse; (4) dilated aortic root may result in AR and LV overload; (5) aortic dissection is a common complication.

Since echocardiographic studies are easily repeatable and can accurately detect the aortic-root dissection and dilatation or both, routine serial measurements of the diameter of the aortic root are feasible. Once the aortic root diameter exceeds 5 cm, more frequent echocardiographic evaluations of root size are required. Because of the high premature mortality, the current practice is to perform prophylactic aortic valve and root replacement once the aortic root diameter exceeds 6 cm [3]. Patient with dissecting hematoma may die from a number of causes secondary to the dissecting hematoma itself, including hemopericardium with cardiac tamponade, occlusion of the coronary ostium as a result of the dissection with subsequent myocardial infarction, or acute AR with progressive refractory congestive heart failure. Echocardiography has been used to identify of patients requiring immediate or delayed surgical correction.

References

1. Simpson LL, Athanassious AM, D'Alton ME. Marfan syndrome in pregnancy. *Curr Opin Obstet Gynecol* 1997;9:337–41.
2. Murdoch JL, Walker BA, Halpern BL, *et al.* Life expectancy and causes of death in the Marfan syndrome. *N Engl J Med* 1972;286:804.
3. McDonald GR, *et al.* Surgical management of patients with the Marfan syndrome and dilatation of the ascending aorta. *J Thorac Cardiovasc Surg* 1981;81:180.

46 Atrioventricular Septal Defect

Jing Ping Sun[1] & James D. Thomas[2]
[1] Emory University School of Medicine; Emory University Hospital Midtown, Atlanta, GA, USA
[2] The Cleveland Clinic Foundation, Cleveland, OH, USA

History

A 2-month-old female has a history of dyspnea, lack of appetite, and cyanosis of the lips and skin since birth.

Echocardiography

The parasternal long axis view shows atrioventricular septal defect in the interchoordal space (Figure 46.1).

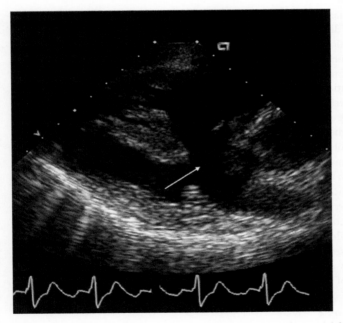

Figure 46.1. The parasternal long axis view shows the atrioventricular septal defect in the interchordal space (arrow).

Practical Handbook of Echocardiography 1st edition. Edited by Jing Ping Sun, Joel Felner and John Merlino. © 2010 Blackwell Publishing Ltd.

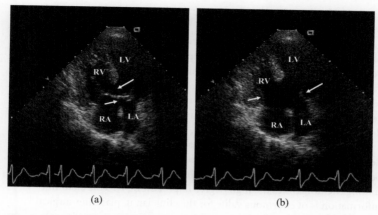

(a)   (b)

Figure 46.2. The apical 4-chamber views show: There is a large hole in the center of the heart. It's located where the septum between the atrial chambers joins the wall between the ventricular chambers (arrows) (A). The common atrioventricular defect is seen spanning the large defect in the atrioventricular septum; the arrows point the leaflets of common valve (B). LA, left atrium; LV, left ventricle; RA, right atrium; RV, right ventricle.

The apical 4-chamber echocardiographic images show: There is a large hole in the center of the heart. It's located where the septum between the atrial chambers joins the wall between the ventricular chambers (arrows) (A). The common atrioventricular defect is seen spanning the large defect in the atrioventricular septum; the arrows point the leaflets of common valve (Figure 46.2).

The left to right shunt and right side regurgitation are detected by color Doppler from parasternal long axis and apical 4-chamber views (Videoclip 46.1).

Discussion

Atrioventricular (AV) canal defect is a large hole in the center of the heart. It also may be called atrioventricular canal defect, or endocardial cusion defect and located where the septum between the atrial chambers joins the wall between the ventricular chambers. This septal defect involves both atrial and ventricular chambers. Also, the tricuspid and mitral valves that normally separate the heart's upper and lower chambers. Instead, a single large valve forms that crosses the defect in the wall between the two sides of the heart [1].

Our case had a single, common atrioventricular valve. The shunts were presented in atrial and ventricular level. When there are two atrioventricular valves, the shunt occurs exclusively at the atrial level, such that the defect has traditionally been considered to be an ostium primum. However, these hearts have been shown to have structural deficiencies of the atrioventricular septa more than of the atrial septa. This concept is supported by the existence of anatomic specimens with this heart defect without ostium primum defects [2].

Echocardiography has provided precise images of the anatomic findings of this congenital malformation with details of the atrioventricular septal defect, the common atrioventricular valve or two separate atrioventricular valves, the relationships between the leaflets of the valves in both forms, septal structures and their defects, disproportion between the left ventricular inflow and outflow tracts, unwedged aorta and the shunts that determine the clinical presentation [3].

Espinola-Zavaleta *et al.* studied 34 patients with atrioventricular septal defect and indicated that the anatomoechocardiographic correlation between specimen hearts and echocardiograms of patients with equivalent findings demonstrates the high degree of precision [4]. This anatomic information is of enormous value for the clinician in planning surgical treatment.

References

1. Mahle WT, Shirali GS, Anderson RH. Echo-morphological correlates in patients with atrioventricular septal defect and common atrioventricular function. *Cardiol Young* 2006;16:43–51.
2. Anderson RH, Ho SY, Falcao L, *et al.* The diagnostic features of atrioventricular septal defect with common atrioventricular junction. *Cardiol Young* 1998;8:33–49.
3. Penkoske PA, Neches W, Anderson RH, Zuberbuhler E. Further observations on the morphology of atrioventricular septal defects. *J Thorac Cardiovasc Surg* 1985;90:611–22.
4. Espinola-Zavaleta N, Muñoz-Castellanos L, Kuri-Nivón M, Keirns C. Understanding atrioventricular septal defect: anatomoechocardiographic correlation. *Cardiovasc Ultrasound* 2008;24:6–33.

47 Cantrell's Syndrome

Yunhua Gao[1], Yali Xu[1] & Xing Sheng Yang[2]
[1]The Third Military Medical University; XinQiao Hospital, ChongQing, China
[2]Emory University School of Medicine; Emory University Hospital Midtown, Atlanta, GA, USA

Case History

A newborn male was admitted due to a pulsating mass of the abdominal wall.

Physical Examination

The patient was mildly cyanotic and crying. There was a pulsating purple mass in the upper abdomen. The diameter of the mass was approximately 4 cm and distended further with crying.

Laboratory

A chest X-ray showed dextrocardia with a thoracic malformation.

Echocardiography revealed the abdominal mass was part of the heart under 1–2 mm of skin. Multiple intracardiac abnormalities were noted (Figure 47.1a). The patient had a complete atrioventricular canal defect (Figure 47.1b, Videoclip 47.1) with a single atrioventricular valve. Both the aorta and pulmonary artery originated from the left ventricle (LV). Continuous wave Doppler across the pulmonic valve revealed a peak velocity of 391 cm/sec, consistent with pulmonary stenosis (Figure 47.2a). Muscular stenosis of the entrance of inferior vena cava was also detected (Figure 47.2b). At 5 months, the patient underwent surgery which demonstrated the dextracardia noted on two-dimensional echocardiography. A left ventricular diverticulum extending into the abdomen through a diaphragmatic hernia terminating at the umbilicus in a omphalocele was also found. Due to inadequate space in the patient's thorax and the complex nature of the congenital abnormality, the surgeon chose to close the abdominal wall without revision of the congenital defects.

Practical Handbook of Echocardiography 1st edition. Edited by Jing Ping Sun, Joel Felner and John Merlino. © 2010 Blackwell Publishing Ltd.

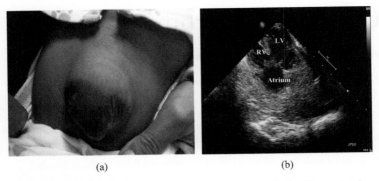

(a)   (b)

Figure 47.1. A pulsating purple mass in the upper abdomen under the skin associated with abdomen wall defect (a). Apical 4-chamber view demonstrates a completed atrioventricular canal malformation: atrial septum defect and common atrioventricular valve (b). LV, left ventricle; RV, right ventricle.

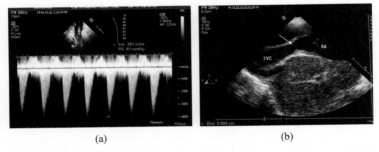

(a)   (b)

Figure 47.2. Continuous wave Doppler across the pulmonic valve revealed a peak velocity of 391 cm/sec, consistent with pulmonary stenosis (a). Muscular stenosis of the entrance of inferior vena cava was also detected (b). IVC, inferior vena cava; RA, right atrium.

Discussion

Cantrell's syndrome was first described in detail by Cantrell *et al.* in 1958 as part of a pentalogy [1]. It is a rare congenital cardiac malformation usually detected in childhood with an incidence of approximately 1 in 65000. The classic clinical picture consists of a combination of abdominal wall defect, and diaphragmatic defect in the sternum as well as absence of the inferior pericardial membrane. Cardiac defects, most often Tetralogy of Fallot or a diverticulum of the LV are commonly noted. In some cases, surgical resection of the left ventricular diverticulum is indicated due to the risk of incarceration of the diverticulum by the diaphragmatic hernia [2].

Prognosis depends on the severity of the cardiac and associated malformations. Most patients die in infancy with very few surviving into adulthood [3].

References

1. Cantrell JR, Haller JA, Ravitch MM. A syndrome of congenital defects involving the abdominal wall, sternum, diaphragm, pericardium and heart. *Surg Gynecol Obstet* 1958;107:602–14.
2. Bernardo SD, Sekarski N, Meijiboom E. Left ventricular diverticulum in a neonate with Cantrell syndrome. *Heart* 2004;90:1320–23.
3. Gruberg L, Goldstein SA, Pfister AJ, *et al.* Cantrell's syndrome – left ventricular diverticulum in an adult patient. *Circulation* 2000;101:109–13.

48 Tetralogy of Fallot with Pulmonary Atresia

Jing Ping Sun, Xing Sheng Yang, Robert D. O'Donnell & John D. Merlino

Emory University School of Medicine; Emory University Hospital Midtown, Atlanta, GA, USA

History

A 30-year-old male was admitted with complaint of exertional shortness of breath, wheezing, and leg swelling of 3 months' duration. He has a history of congenital heart disease and has hemoptysis for 2–3 years.

Physical Examination

He was mildly cyanosed and clubbed with pectus carinatum. Blood pressure was 126/78 mmHg. Cardiac examination revealed a grade 2/6 systolic heart murmur which was heard throughout the precordium.

Laboratory

Electrocardiography confirmed sinus tachycardia with first-degree atrial ventricular block, biatrial enlargement, right ventricular hypertrophy (RVH), incomplete right bundle branch block, ST-T and T-wave abnormalities diffusely. Chest X-ray revealed that the cardiac silhouette was markedly enlarged and there appeared to be a right-sided aortic arch. There was significant vascular congestion in both hilar regions.

Echocardiography revealed: ventricular septal defect (VSD) is typically located in the perimembranous region with a left to right shunt of 2.12 m/sec. Placement of the aorta shifted toward the right (overriding aorta), RVH, well contracting left ventricle (LV), atria dilated, no identifiable main pulmonary artery pulmonary atresia (Figure 48.1, Videoclip 48.1). Transthoracic suprasternal view shows aortic arch and one right pulmonary artery derived from descending aorta (located in right side) (Figure 48.2). The peak velocity of tricuspid regurgitation (TR) was 546 cm/sec, and the gradient was 119 mmHg.

Magnetic resonance imaging showed: there are three right pulmonary arteries (RPA 1, 2, 3) derived from descending aorta, and a left sidedplexus of arteries (plexus) derived from left subclavian artery. The left lung is smaller than right due to short of blood supply (Figure 48.3). A hypoplasia

Practical Handbook of Echocardiography 1st edition. Edited by Jing Ping Sun, Joel Felner and John Merlino. © 2010 Blackwell Publishing Ltd.

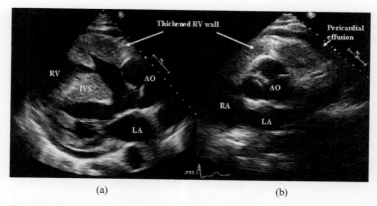

(a)   (b)

Figure 48.1. Transthoracic echocardiography: parasternal long-axis view shows right ventricular hypertrophy, ventricular septal defect and overriding of the septum by the large aorta (a). Parasternal short-axis view shows that the pulmonary artery is absent, small amount of pericardial effusion can be seen (b). AO, aorta; IVS, interventricular septum; LA, left atrium; RA, right atrium; RV, right ventricle.

of left lung and plexus of vessels which originates from the left subclavian and supplies collaterals to the arterial circulation of the left lung, and demonstrated those findings by echocardiography (Figure 48.2), indicating the presence of tetralogy of Fallot (TOF) with pulmonary atresia. The ascending aorta was dilated. The descending aorta was on the right and passed posterior to the left atrium. The left brachiocephalic vein passed posterior to the ascending aorta to join the superior vena cava. The LV was mildly dilated with moderately reduced systolic function. There was mild

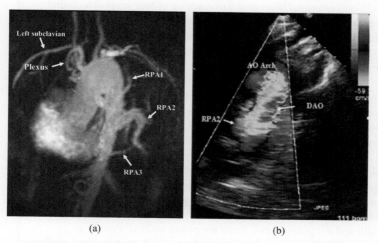

(a)   (b)

Figure 48.2. MRI image show that there are three right pulmonary arteries (RPA 1, 2, 3) derived from descending aorta, and a left sided plexus of arteries (plexus) derived from left subclavian artery (A). Transthoracic super sternal view shows aortic arch and one right pulmonary artery derived from descending aorta (located in right side) (B). These two images are comparable.

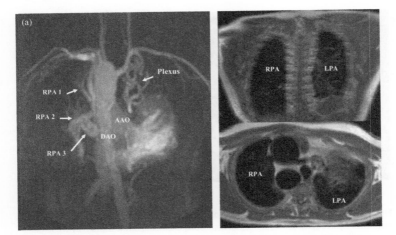

Figure 48.3. MRI image shows that there are three right pulmonary arteries (RPA 1, 2, 3) derived from descending aorta, and a left sidedplexus of arteries (plexus) derived from left subclavian artery (a). The left lung is smaller than right due to short of blood supply (b and c). AAO, ascending aorta; DAO, descending aorta; LPA, left pulmonary artery; RPA, right pulmonary artery.

AR. The RV was severely dilated with severely reduced systolic function. There was moderate TR.

Discussion

TOF is a congenital heart problem made up of four heart defects that occur together, including ventriculoseptal defect, pulmonary infundibular stenosis, shifting of the aorta toward the right (overriding aorta) and RVH.

Few patients with TOF reach adulthood with an average life expectancy of 12 years without surgery.

Pulmonary atresia with VSD is considered the extreme end of the anatomic spectrum of TOF. TOF with pulmonary atresia (TOF-PA) is worthy of separate consideration. Because of the wide variability of pulmonary blood supply, diagnosis and surgical management of TOF-PA is more difficult than that of classic TOF [1].

Anatomy of the pulmonary arteries and the source of pulmonary artery blood supply may widely vary in TOF-PA. Persistence of descending thoracic branches accounts for the abnormal pulmonary arterial supply, such as our case. Major aortopulmonary collateral arteries may anastomose at any site in the pulmonary vascular tree. Most often, the right and left pulmonary arteries are patent and maintain free communication with each other, in which case they are termed confluent pulmonary arteries. Also the pulmonary arteries may be hypoplastic and nonconfluent. No antegrade blood flow is present from the RV to the pulmonary arteries. Generally the PDA is an important source of blood supply, although occasionally it is absent [2].

Rare sources of pulmonary blood flow include an aortopulmonary window, a persistent fifth aortic arch, and coronary-to-pulmonary artery fistulae. Identification of the pulmonary arterial supply is essential in planning the type of surgical repair.

Aortopulmonary collaterals most frequently arise from the descending aorta, as in our case, and vary in number from two to six. In some cases, the collaterals may arise from the brachiocephalic arteries, but rarely, from the coronary arteries.

References

1. Tchervenkov CI, Roy N. Congenital heart surgery nomenclature and database project: pulmonary atresia–ventricular septal defect. *Ann Thorac Surg* 2000;69(4 Suppl.):S97–105.
2. Van Praagh R, Van Praagh S, Nebesar RA, *et al.* Tetralogy of Fallot: underdevelopment of the pulmonary infundibulum and its sequelae. *Am J Cardiol* 1970;26:25–33.

49 Coarctation of the Aorta

Joel M. Felner[1] & Jing Ping Sun[2]

[1]Grady Memorial Hospital; Emory University School of Medicine, Atlanta, GA, USA
[2]Emory University School of Medicine; Emory University Hospital Midtown, Atlanta, GA, USA

History

A 30-year-old male complains of leg fatigue and dyspnea on exertion. He has an 8-year history of hypertension.

Physical Examination

The temperature was 37.2°C and pulse was 88 and regular; blood pressure was 168/92 mmHg and respiration rate was 20/minute. S4 gallop at the apex was noted on auscultation. Systolic murmur was heard along the left heart border. Peripheral pulses—femoral pulses are 1+ bilaterally and delayed when simultaneously compared with the radial pulses.

Laboratory

Two-dimensional echocardiography: moderate–severe left ventricular hypertrophy (LVH) (Figure 49.1) with normal systolic function and diastolic dysfunction type 2 (pseudonormal pattern). The suprasternal window shows a discrete area of narrowing within the lumen of the thoracic aorta. Color Doppler image shows turbulence in the arch due to the coarctation (Figure 49.2a and Videoclip 49.1a). The echocardiographic images are comparable with angiogram and magnetic resonance imaging (Videoclip 49.1).

Continuous wave Doppler determines the severity by obtaining maximal flow velocities across the narrowed area and calculating the pressure gradient (56 mmHg) across the coarctation (Figure 49.3). This patient also has a bicuspid aortic valve as demonstrated by transesophageal echocardiography at angle 62° (Figure 49.4). Electrocardiogram: normal sinus rhythm with evidence of LVH. Chest X-ray results: (1) rib notching; (2) normal cardiopericardial silhouette; and (3) normal lung fields.

Aortogram after injection of contrast into the aortic root demonstrates marked focal narrowing of the proximal descending thoracic aorta. The angiogram shows coarctation of the aorta distal to the left subclavian

Practical Handbook of Echocardiography 1st edition. Edited by Jing Ping Sun,
Joel Felner and John Merlino. © 2010 Blackwell Publishing Ltd.

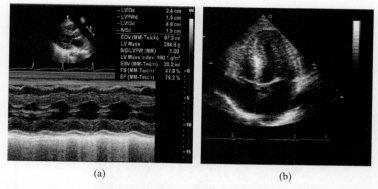

(a)   (b)

Figure 49.1. Two-dimensional and M-mode echocardiography demonstrated a patient with moderate–severe left ventricular hypertrophy (a and b).

(Figure 49.2b and Videoclip 49.2). Magnetic resonance images also show the coarctation of the thoracic aorta (Figure 49.2c).

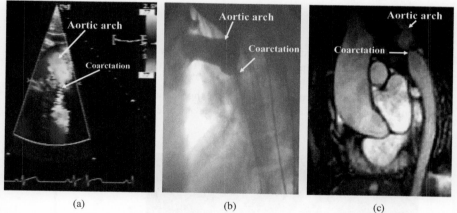

(a)   (b)   (c)

Figure 49.2. Transthoracic echocardiography: suprasternal view shows a discrete area of narrowing within the lumen of the thoracic aorta. Color Doppler image shows turbulence in the arch due to the coarctation (a). Aortic angiogram shows coarctation of thoracic aorta (b). Magnetic resonance imaging shows coarctation of thoracic aorta (c). Three different cardiac images are comparable.

Discussion

In a patient with coarctation of the aorta, the carotid and upper extremity pulses are normal to slightly enhanced in upstroke. The femoral pulse is diminished and also delayed in onset compared to the radial pulse. The lower extremity blood pressure in this patient was 120/80, i.e., significantly

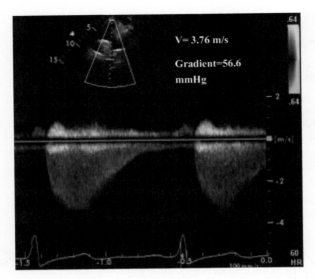

Figure 49.3. Continuous wave Doppler determines the severity by obtaining maximal flow velocities across the narrowed area and calculating the pressure gradient (56 mmHg) across the coarctation.

lower than the upper extremities, which are normally higher. These findings are all consistent with coarctation of the aorta beyond the origin of the left subclavian artery.

Coarctation may occur at any level of the thoracic aorta, but it is most commonly (95 % of cases) located left subclavian artery near the

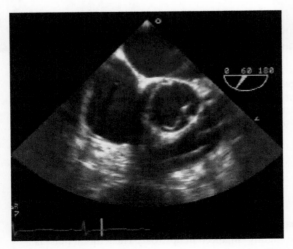

Figure 49.4. This patient also has a bicuspid aortic valve demonstrated by transesophageal echocardiography at an angle of 62°.

ligamentum arteriosum [1]. A bicuspid aortic valve is found in between 40 and 80 % of patients with isolated coarctation of the post-ductal type. Coarctation is also the most common cardiac anomaly associated with Turner's syndrome [2]. The most common noncardiac abnormality is intracerebral aneurysm. Unless very severe, coarctation frequently is asymptomatic until the mid-teens, and even then is commonly diagnosed by finding hypertension or an abnormal chest X-ray. These patients are at increased risk for infective endocarditis.

Aortic coarctation causes severe obstruction of blood flow in the descending thoracic aorta. As a result, the descending aorta and its branches are perfused by collateral channels from the axillary and internal thoracic arteries through the intercostal arteries.

The anatomical findings are the result of thickening of the media of the aortic wall resulting in a ridge or shelf.

Pathophysiologically there is a left ventricular outflow tract gradient across the coarctation that causes hypertension in proximal vessels and hypotension in the distal vessels. This increased afterload leads to LVH and eventually congestive heart failure. Proximal hypertension can lead to early cardiovascular disease if uncorrected.

Surgery was recommended to remedy this patient's hypertension and prevent its complications. The optimal time for operation should be between 2 and 6 years of age. If surgery is delayed, some patients will remain hypertensive despite successful anatomical surgical correction. Some patients with coarctation of the aorta may be treated by intravascular balloon dilation via femoral artery catheterization or have an endocardial repair [3].

Treatment indications include (1) decrease in lumen diameter by >50% at site of coarctation and (2) gradient of >20 mmHg across lesion [4].

References

1. Abbruzzese PA, Aidala E. Aortic coarctation: an overview. *J Cardiovasc Med* 2007;8(2):123–8.
2. Nora JJ, Torres FG, Sinha AK, McNamara DG. Characteristic cardiovascular anomalies of XO Turner syndrome, XX and XY phenotype and XO-XX Turner mosaic. *Am J Cardiol.* 1970;25(6):639–41.
3. Carr JA. The results of catheter-based therapy compared with surgical repair of adult aortic coarctation. *J Am Coll Cardiol* 2006, 21;47(6):1101–7.
4. Anagnostopoulos-Tzifa A. Management of aortic coarctation in adults: endovascular versus surgical therapy. *Hellenic J Cardiol* 2007;48(5):290–95.

50 Supravalvular Aortic Stenosis with Williams Syndrome

Jing Ping Sun[1], Xing Sheng Yang[1] & Joel M. Felner[2]
[1] Emory University School of Medicine; Emory University Hospital Midtown, Atlanta, GA, USA
[2] Grady Memorial Hospital; Emory University School of Medicine, Atlanta, GA, USA

History

A 20-year-old male with history of Williams syndrome and supravalvular aortic valve stenosis (AS). The patient was referred for surgical evaluation.

Physical Examination

The blood pressure was 110/80 mmHg and the heart rate was 138/minute; auscultation revealed a grade 3/6 jet systolic murmur at the aortic area.

Laboratory

Angiogram showed supravalvular AS.

Echocardiography: The left ventricle was normal in size and function (ejection fraction = 75%). The aortic valve was normal. Parasternal long-axis recording found a diffuse area of supravalvular narrowing (hourglass lesion). Compared with the part of aortic sinus and ascending aorta (above the lesion), the diameter of narrow part is significantly small (Figure 50.1a). Angiogram shows the similarity of the actual anatomic lesion of supravalvular aortic stenosis (SVAS) (Figure 50.1b).

Transesophageal echocardiography (TEE) recording at angle 131° illustrates a diffuse area of supravalvular narrowing (hourglass lesion) with a superimposed membrane. The color Doppler recording shows the blood flow through the narrow part with high velocity (400 cm/sec; gradient is 64 mmHg) from apical 5-chamber view (Figure 50.2, Videoclip 50.1).

Three-dimensional TEE recording at angle 180° (aortic short view above aortic valve) illustrates diffuse area of supravalvular narrowing with a superimposed membrane (Videoclip 50.2).

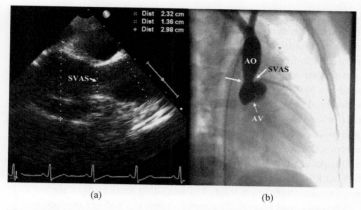

(a)   (b)

Figure 50.1. Parasternal long-axis view illustrates a diffuse area of supravalvular narrowing (hourglass lesion). Compared with the part of aortic sinus and atrial septal defect (above the lesion), the diameter of narrowed part is significantly small (a). Angiogram shows the similarity of the actual anatomic lesion of supravalvular aortic valve stenosis (arrows) (b). AV, aortic valve; SVAS, supravalvular aortic valve stenosis.

Hospital Course

He underwent surgical procedure without complications. He was discharged in stable condition.

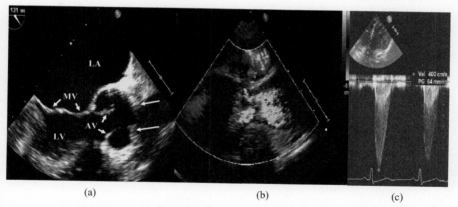

(a)   (b)   (c)

Figure 50.2. Transesophageal echocardiography recording at an angle of 131° illustrates a diffuse area of supravalvular narrowing (hourglass lesion) with a superimposed membrane (long arrows) (a). The color Doppler recording shows the blood flow through the narrow part with high velocity (b). The peak velocity of the flow through the narrow part is 400 cm/sec; gradient is 64 mmHg from apical 5-chamber view (c). AV, aortic valve; LA, left atrium; LV, left ventricle; MV, mitral valve.

Discussion

Approximately half of patients with SVAS have Williams' syndrome, involving increased intestinal calcium absorption and characterized by developmental delay, distinctive facial features, small nails and short stature. Most patients with SVAS, particularly if they have Williams' syndrome, also have evidence of right ventricular outflow tract obstruction.

A reduction in the elasticity of great arteries may lead to an excessive collagen deposition in the aortic media due to increased stress in the artery wall, and to a hypertrophy of smooth muscle cells. Therefore, a circumferential narrowing at the sinotubular aortic junction and an obstructive arteriopathy form that can include aortic arch, major arteries and pulmonary arteries (PAs) [1]. Supravalvular aortic stenosis has two major types: the localized type and the diffuse type. In the localized type, the malformation consists in a supravalvular narrow ring at the aortic sinotubular junction. The diffuse type is a more severe one associated with an anatomical malformation located in ascending aorta (AAO), aortic arch, arch vessels and PAs [2]. The aortic leaflets in SVAS are exposed to a decrease in mobility and a higher pressure, which may lead to accelerated aortic valve degeneration.

Echocardiography reveals circumferential narrowing in the sinotubular aortic junction or hourglass stenosis. Doppler studies are useful to evaluate valvular lesions that may be associated with SVAS [2]. Electrocardiography may reveal myocardial ischemia and left ventricular hypertrophy. Angiography is only necessary when the patient is suspected of having SVAS or pulmonary artery stenosis.

References

1. Ly DY, Brooke B, Davis EC, et al. Elastin is an essential determinant of arterial morphogenesis. *Nature* 1998;393:276–80.
2. Eroglu AG, Babaoglu K, Oztunc F, et al. Echocardiographic follow-up of children with supravalvular aortic stenosis. *Pediatr Cardiol* 2006;27:707–12.

51 Discrete Subaortic Stenosis

Jing Ping Sun[1], Xing Sheng Yang[1] & Joel M. Felner[2]

[1] Emory University School of Medicine; Emory University Hospital Midtown, Atlanta, GA, USA
[2] Grady Memorial Hospital; Emory University School of Medicine, Atlanta, GA, USA

History

A 40-year-old female with history of congenital heart defect repaired at the age of 11. She presented with a 2-month history of shortness of breath on exertion.

Laboratory

Echocardiography: There is mild left ventricular hypertrophy. The left ventricle (LV) is normal in size and function.

There is mild to moderate thickening of the mitral valve with mild MR. The aortic valve (AV) leaflets are thickened with a peak gradient of 32 consistent with mild aortic valve stenosis (AS). There is moderate to severe aortic regurgitation (AR). There is subaortic membrane, which can be well seen in a parasternal long-axis (PLA) and, in particular, in an apical 5-chamber view, because it places the membrane perpendicular to the path of the scan (Figure 51.1).

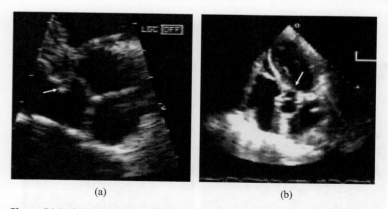

(a) (b)

Figure 51.1. (a) Parasternal long-axis view shows the subaortic membrane (arrow). (b) Apical 5-chamber view is particularly valuable because it places the membrane (arrow) perpendicular to the path of the scan.

Practical Handbook of Echocardiography 1st edition. Edited by Jing Ping Sun, Joel Felner and John Merlino. © 2010 Blackwell Publishing Ltd.

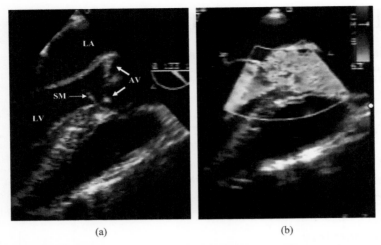

(a)   (b)

Figure 51.2. Transesophageal echocardiogram images indicate a subaortic membrane (arrow) (a), which can be well seen with aortic valve stenosis turbulent flow in left ventricular outflow tract during systole (b). AV, aortic valve; LA, left atrium; LV, left ventricle; SM, subaortic membrane.

TEE images indicate a subaortic membrane, which can be well seen during diastole and systole with turbulent flow in left ventricular outflow tract (LVOT) (Figure 51.2, Videoclip 51.1).

M-mode recording from our case with discrete subaortic stenosis shows the typical early systolic notch followed by high-frequency fluttering of the valve leaflet throughout the remainder of ejection period. Continuous wave Doppler recording indicates high-velocity flow through LVOT (Figure 51.3).

The right ventricular size and function are normal.

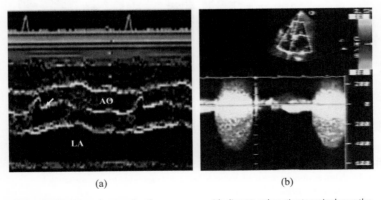

(a)   (b)

Figure 51.3. M-mode recording from our case with discrete subaortic stenosis shows the typical early systolic notch (arrow) followed by high frequency fluttering of the valve leaflet throughout the remainder of ejection period (a). Continuous wave Doppler recording indicates high-velocity flow through left ventricular outflow tract (b). AO, aorta; LA, left atrium.

The tricuspid valve is normal with mild tricuspid regurgitation. This calculates to a systolic pulmonary pressure of approximately 45–50 mmHg.

Discussion

Subvalvular aortic stenosis is the second most common form of AS. Among children with congenital AS, subvalvular AS accounts for 10–14% of cases [1].

Fixed subaortic stenosis is an obstruction of LVOT below the AV. There are three different types: the discrete fixed membranous subaortic stenosis (DMSS), the discrete fixed fibromuscular subaortic stenosis (DFSS), and the tunnel subaortic stenosis (TSS), DFSS and TSS are more frequently severe than membranous subaortic stenosis. Our case represents discrete fixed membranous subaortic stenosis.

Discrete subaortic stenosis is a manifestation of a geometric anatomic alteration in the LVOT. This endocardial abnormality involves not only the subaortic ridge but also the leaflets of the adjacent valves [2]. DSS seems to be acquired, because it is almost never present at birth, and it is believed that the obstruction of LVOT is a consequence of some abnormality of ventricular motion, growth, hypertrophy, combination of factors or additional factors such as inflammatory or genetic [3].

The most common symptom in patients with DSS is diminished exercise tolerance. The major symptom in our case is dyspnea on exertion. Discrete subaortic stenosis is sometimes associated with various other cardiac malformations, such as small or spontaneously closed ventricular septal defect, patent duct arteries, patent foramina ovalia, and the diffuse type of LVOT stenosis [4]. Except for congenital cardiac abnormalities, acquired AR is the most common lesion found in cases with DSS and can be progressive.

Echocardiography in PLA view can reveal LVOT with a discrete subaortic stenosis. The maximal instantaneous gradient across the LVOT was calculated from the peak spectral Doppler velocity using the modified Bernoulli equation [5].

Discrete subaortic stenosis has been treated surgically for many years, but the optimal operative management and the timing of surgery remain controversial. Many studies have suggested surgery for patients who have LV–aorta gradients that exceed 30 mmHg or a coexisting cardiac defect that requires surgical correction [2].

References

1. Kitchiner D, Jackson M, Malaiya N, *et al.* Incidence and prognosis of obstruction of the left ventricular outflow tract in Liverpool (1960–91): a study of 313 patients. *Br Heart J* 1994;71:588.
2. Rayburn ST, Netherland DE, Heath BJ. Discrete membranous subaortic stenosis: improved results after resection and myectomy. *Ann Thorac Surg* 1997;64:105–9.
3. Kuralay E, Ozal E, Bingol H, *et al.* Discrete subaortic stenosis: assessing

adequacy of myectomy by transesophageal echocardiography. *J Card Surg* 1999;14:348–53.

4. Darcin OT, Yagdi T, Atay Y, *et al.* Discrete subaortic stenosis—surgical outcomes and follow-up results. *Tex Heart Inst J* 2003;30:286–92.

5. Feigl A, Feigl D, Lucas RV, Jr, *et al.* Involvement of the aortic valve cusps in discrete subaortic stenosis. *Pediatr Cardiol* 1984;5:185–9.

52 Cor Triatriatum Sinister

Jing Ping Sun[1], Xing Sheng Yang[1] & Joel M. Felner[2]
[1] Emory University School of Medicine; Emory University Hospital Midtown, Atlanta, GA, USA
[2] Grady Memorial Hospital; Emory University School of Medicine, Atlanta, GA, USA

History

A 20-year-old male admitted with a 2-week history of palpitations and right-sided chest discomfort.

Physical Examination

Heart rate was 92 beats/minute. No significant heart murmur heard.

Laboratory

Electrocardiogram confirmed the presence of frequent atrial premature beats.

Transthoracic echocardiography: parasternal long-axis (PLA) view shows a membrane dividing left atrium (LA) into two chambers The M-mode of PLA view shows a membrane dividing LA into two parts. An apical 2-chamber view shows a membrane dividing LA into upper and lower chambers. Transesophageal echocardiography apical 4-chamber view shows a clear membrane dividing LA into two chambers (Figure 52.1, Videoclip 52.1).

Discussion

Cor triatriatum is a congenital cardiac abnormality with three atria, first reported in 1868 [1]. It is found in 0.1% of cases with congenital heart disease [2]. In cor triatriatum, the atrium is divided into two parts by a fold of tissue, a membrane, or a fibromuscular band; which can occur in LA, named cor triatriatum sinistrum. This can occur in right atrium (cor triatriatum dextrum). The classical cor triatriatum in LA is divided into two chambers by a fibromuscular membrane: a posterosuperior chamber receiving the pulmonary veins, and an anteroinferior chamber (true left atrium) contacts with the mitral valve and contains the atrial appendage and true atrial septum that bears fossa ovalis [3].

Practical Handbook of Echocardiography 1st edition. Edited by Jing Ping Sun,
Joel Felner and John Merlino. © 2010 Blackwell Publishing Ltd.

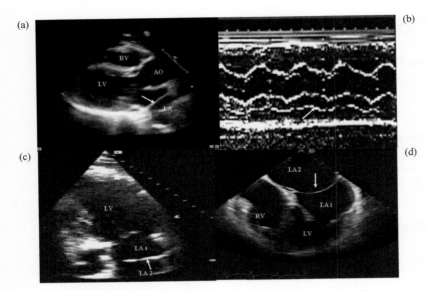

Figure 52.1. Transthoracic echocardiography: parasternal long-axis view shows a membrane (arrow) dividing left atrium into two chambers (a). The M-mode of parasternal long-axis view shows a membrane (arrow) dividing left atrium into two parts (b). An apical 2-chamber view shows a membrane (arrow) dividing left atrium into upper and lower chambers (c). Transesophageal echocardiography apical 4-chamber view shows a clear membrane (arrow) dividing left atrium into two chambers (d). AO, aorta; LA, left atrium; LV, left ventricle; RV, right ventricle.

In adult populational cor triatriatum is frequently an isolated finding, such as in our case. In children, this abnormality may be associated with some congenital cardiac lesions such as tetralogy of Fallot, ventricular septal defect, atrioventricular septal defect, double outlet right ventricle , coarctation of the aorta, partial anomalous pulmonary venous connection, persistent left superior vena cava with unroofed coronary sinus, and common atrioventricular canal. Rarely, asplenia or polysplenia has been reported in these patients [4].

Complete surgical resection of the membrane and closure of the atrial septum with a pericardial patch is a common approach. The outcome is excellent in adults with isolated cor triatriatum [4].

References

1. Church WS. Congenital malformation of the heart: abnormal septum in the left auricle. *Trans Pathol Soc Lond* 1868;19:188–90.
2. Van Son JAM, Danielson GK, Schaff HV, *et al.* Cor triatriatum: diagnosis, operative approach and late results. *Mayo Clin Proc* 1993;68:854–9.
3. Rorie M, Xie GY, Miles H, *et al.* Diagnosis and surgical correction of cor triatriatum in an adult: combined use of transesophageal echocardiography and catheterization. *Cathet Cardiovasc Interv* 2000;51:83–6.
4. Shirani J, Kalyansundaram A, Pourmoghadam KK, *et al.* Cor triatriatum. EMedicine. (Updated: September 18, 2008).

Part 8
Cardiac Tumor

53 Inferior Vena Caval Masses

Jing Ping Sun[1], William J. Stewart[2] & James D. Thomas[2]

[1] Emory University School of Medicine; Emory University Hospital Midtown, Atlanta, GA, USA
[2] The Cleveland Clinic Foundation, Cleveland, OH, USA

Detection of inferior vena cava (IVC) masses has important clinical implications for the management of patients with retroperitoneal or metastatic tumors and migratory thrombi. Due to the direct connection between the renal vein and IVC, renal carcinoma is a well-recognized cause of IVC mass. Because surgical resection may be curative for many patients with renal carcinoma without metastasis, the presence of IVC involvement should be searched for preoperatively. We have reported on the use of echocardiography to evaluate the IVC before surgical resection of solid organ tumors in 62 patients.

Studied Cases

Transthoracic echocardiography (TTE) or transesophageal echocardiography (TEE) demonstrated IVC involvement in 56 of 62 patients (90%). The metastatic mass can be clearly outlined by echocardiography. A mass in IVC, which has metastasized from renal carcinoma, is shown in Figure 53.1a, Videoclip 53.1a; and a metastatic mass to right atrium (RA) is shown in Figure 53.1b and Videoclip 53.1b. TTE and TEE underestimated the level of IVC involvement in three patients with a level II mass (one failed by transthoracic, one failed by transesophageal, and one by TTE and TEE).

Discussion

Previous studies have reported that the most common causes of IVC masses include hypernephroma, hepatoma, Wilm's tumor, lymphosarcoma, and leiomyosarcoma [1]. Our study found a similar distribution of etiologies with renal cell carcinoma being by far the most prevalent tumor in this setting. Generally, these tumors invade IVC through direct hematogenous extension, which explains the high proportion of abdominal and retroperitoneal sources. Although a mass may result in partial or total obstruction of IVC, the most common manifestation is pulmonary embolization [2]. Often, these emboli may not be clinically apparent and may be detected only by ventilation and/or perfusion scanning, pulmonary angiography, or occasionally by directly

Practical Handbook of Echocardiography 1st edition. Edited by Jing Ping Sun, Joel Felner and John Merlino. © 2010 Blackwell Publishing Ltd.

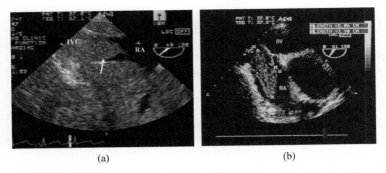

(a)   (b)

Figure 53.1. Mass in inferior vena cava (arrow), metastasized from renal carcinoma in one case (a). Mass in right atrium in another case with renal carcinoma (b). IVC, inferior vena cava; RA, right atrium; RV, right ventricle. Reproduced with permission from Elsevier.

visualizing their passage through the inferior vena cava, right heart chambers, and pulmonary artery by echocardiography.

Preoperative imaging studies are essential to the determination of the presence and distal limits of an IVC mass. This provides important information with regards to the surgical approach for their removal.

Contrast inferior venacavography, although the gold standard with respect to accuracy, is invasive and associated with complications, such as dye-induced renal dysfunction. TTE is a reliable and convenient tool for evaluating cardiac sources of embolism. It should be used as a preoperative test. The subcostal view is part of a routine TTE study. It enables accurate evaluation of the proximal IVC as it extends into RA. This view is used to screen for IVC masses and to assess RA pressure. Compared with operative findings, TTE detected and localized IVC masses with a diagnostic accuracy of 90%, supporting the use of TTE as an effective screening modality. The additional advantages of TEE compared with TTE have been previously described, including the opportunity to use higher frequency transducers with less obstructed views [3].

References

1. Weyman AE. *Principle and Practice of Echocardiography*, 2nd edition. Philadelphia: Lee and Febiger, 1994, p. 854.
2. Van Kuyk M, Mols P, Englert M. Right atrial thrombus leading to pulmonary embolism. *Br Heart J* 1984;51:462–4.
3. Marshall VF, Middleton RG, Holswade GR, Goldsmith EI. Surgery for renal cell carcinoma in the vena cava. *J Urol* 1970;103:414–20.

54 The Right Ventricular Capillary Hemangiomas with Cystic Change

Yunhua Gao[1], Pin Qian[1] & Jing Ping Sun[2]
[1]The Third Military Medical University; XinQiao Hospital, ChongQing, China
[2]Emory University School of Medicine; Emory University Hospital Midtown, Atlanta, GA, USA

History

A 20-year old male presented with a 3-month history of heart murmur and shortness of breath.

Laboratory

Transthoracic echocardiography (TTE) in parasternal long-axis and short-axis (PSA) views showed a mass in the right ventricular outflow tract (RVOT). The mass was an elliptic type with a clear high echo density boundary. The echo density was decreased at the center of the mass (Figure 54.1). A stalk was 0.65 cm in length, which connected the mass to the ventricular septum. The area of the mass was 4.0×2.8 cm^2. The shape of mass was slightly changed during the cardiac cycle (Videoclip 54.1).

The RVOT was blocked by this mass, with a high-velocity flow demonstrated by color Doppler (Figure 54.1b and Videoclip 54.1b,c). The flow velocity was 3.1 m/sec by continuous wave Doppler (gradient 46.5 mmHg). The velocity of diastolic flow in the proximal end of the stalk attached to the septum was 1.1 m/sec.

TTE: apical 4-chamber view showed that right atrium (RA) and right ventricle (RV) were enlarged. There was mild tricuspid regurgitation; the peak regurgitant velocity was 4.2 m/sec, suggesting RV systolic pressure >65 mmHg.

Hospital Course

The tumor was successfully removed surgically. The pathologic diagnosis was right ventricular capillary hemangiomas with cystic change. The patient was discharged in good conditions.

Practical Handbook of Echocardiography 1st edition. Edited by Jing Ping Sun, Joel Felner and John Merlino. © 2010 Blackwell Publishing Ltd.

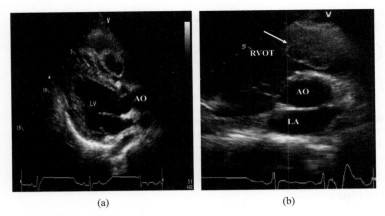

(a)   (b)

Figure 54.1. Parasternal long-axis view shows a mass (arrow) in the right ventricular outflow tract. The mass is an elliptic type with a clear high echo density boundary and a stalk. The echo density is decreased at the center of the mass (a). The parasternal short-axis view shows a mass (arrow) almost blocking the right ventricular outflow tract (b). AO, aorta; LA, left atrium; LV, left ventricle; RVOT, right ventricular outflow tract.

Discussion

Primary cardiac tumors are extremely rare, with an incidence of 1.7 per 100,000 cases at autopsy [1]. The majority (75%) of primary cardiac tumors are benign, and they can arise from any layer of the heart (pericardium, myocardium, or endocardium [2]. Cardiac hemangiomas (including capillary, venous, racemose, and cavernous histological subtypes) occur in all ages, with a slight male predominance. Subendocardial hemangiomas have been described in all the cardiac chambers, but most occur on the right side of the heart and left atrium (LA) [3].

Clinical manifestations are dependent upon tumor location. A tumor developing in the pericardium can produce pericardial effusion, hemopericardium, and even lethal tamponade [2]. An RA hemangioma on the rim of the foramen ovale or interatrial septum can mimic atrial myxoma, with associated tumor emboli or superior vena cava obstruction. When situated at the right side of the interventricular septum, the hemangioma may simulate infundibular pulmonary stenosis. The patient may present with congestive heart failure (CHF), usually right sided, due to restricted filling [4,3]. Hemangioma of RV can cause outflow tract obstruction. This case had RA and RV enlargement and the symptoms of heart failure caused by RVOT obstruction and secondary high RV pressure.

References

1. Strauss R, Merliss R. Primary tumors of the heart. *Arch Pathol* 1945;39:74–8.
2. Silber EN. *Heart Disease.* 2nd edition. New York: Macmillan, 1987, pp. 1427–48.

3. Tabry IF, Nassar VH, Rizk G, *et al.* Cavernous hemangioma of the heart: case report and review of the literature. *J Thorac Cardiovasc Surg* 1975;69:415–20.
4. Soberman MS. Hemangioma of the right ventricle causing outflow tract obstruction. *J Cardiovasc Surg* 1988;96:307–9.

55 Cardiac Lipoma

Jing Ping Sun, Xing Sheng Yang, Dale Yoo & John D. Merlino

Emory University School of Medicine; Emory University Hospital Midtown, Atlanta, GA, USA

History

A 29-year-old female with inferolateral T wave abnormalities on electrocardiogram while on routine physical exam.

Laboratory

Echocardiogram: Apical 4-, 2-, and 3-chamber views show a well-circumscribed mass measuring 3.0×2.7 cm^2 in the posterolateral wall of left ventricle (LV) (Figure 55.1, Videoclip 55.1 and 55.2). The remaining cardiac structure and function were normal.

Magnetic resonance imaging (MRI) revealed complete suppression of the mass with fat saturation pulsation, suggesting an intramyocardial lipoma in the posterolateral wall of LV.

Repeat imaging every 6–8 months was obtained. Nearly four years later, transthoracic echocardiography was performed and measured the LV lipoma near the apex which was similar in size to previous measurements. Since the patient was not symptomatic, surgery was not recommended.

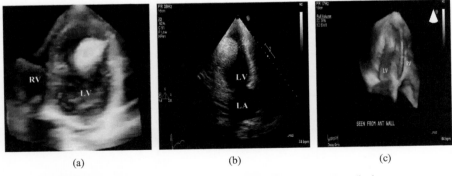

(a) (b) (c)

Figure 55.1. (a–c) Apical 4-, 2-, and 3-chamber views show a well-circumscribed mass measuring 3.0 cm × 2.7 cm^2 in the posterolateral wall of left ventricle. LA, left atrium; LV, left ventricle; RV, right ventricle.

Practical Handbook of Echocardiography 1st edition. Edited by Jing Ping Sun, Joel Felner and John Merlino. © 2010 Blackwell Publishing Ltd.

Discussion

Cardiac lipomas (CLPs) are extremely rare benign tumors composed of adipose tissue. These tumors can develop on the pericardial surface or inside the cardiac chambers [1]. Usually lipomas remain asymptomatic, and are generally incidentally detected on echocardiograms performed for other reasons. An extremely rare type of lipoma, usually associated with tuberous sclerosis, occurs in children and causes thickening of the myocardial wall with narrowing of the cardiac cavity [2].

Fibromas are usually located in the ventricle (LV ≥ RV), interventricular septum, or RA. The symptoms in patients with ventriculoseptal involvement may include heart failure, arrhythmias, sudden death, cyanosis and chest pain [2]. Typical echocardiographic features of a lipoma include attachment along the atrial or ventricular septum, hyper-refractile quality relative to the myocardium, a sessile and well-circumscribed nature [3]. Computed tomography and MRI are the useful tools for diagnosis of lipoma. The diagnosis is ultimately confirmed with pathological examination. Usually, the tumors are successfully removed, and the prognosis is excellent [4].

We report a case with a cardiac lipoma in LV posterolateral wall near the apex. The patient is asymptomatic because the tumor does not interfere with cardiac function or regular flow.

References

1. Grande AM, Minzioni G, Pederzolli C, *et al.* Cardiac lipomas. Description of 3 cases. *J Cardiovasc Surg (Torino)* 1998;39:813–5.
2. Ozaki N, Mukohara N, Yoshida M, *et al.* Cardiac lipoma in the ventricular septum—a case report. *Thorac Cardiovasc Surg* 2006;54:356–7.
3. Chen MS, Sun JP, Asher CR. A right atrial mass and a pseudomass. *Echocardiography* 2005;22:441–5.
4. Yano H, Konagai N, Maeda M, *et al.* Right atrial lipoma with calcification in ascending aorta: report of a case. *Kyobu Geka* 2002;55:1057–60.

56 Hemangioma in the Right Ventricle

Hong Tang[1], Jing Ping Sun[2] & Xing Sheng Yang[2]

[1] Sichuan University, Chengdu, Sichuan, China
[2] Emory University School of Medicine; Emory University Hospital Midtown, Atlanta, GA, USA

History

A 50-year old male was admitted with chest pain for 15 days.

Physical Examination

Blood pressure was 122/78 mm Hg; heart rate was regular (80/minute).
Cardiac examination revealed grade 3/6 systolic murmur heard at the sternal border.

Laboratory

Transthoracic echocardiography: parasternal short-axis view reveals a 6 × 4 cm² mass in the right ventricular outflow tract, and apical 4-chamber view shows the mass in right ventricle (RV) apex. This mass has a clear boundary and a stalk attached to lower part of anteroseptum (Figure 56.1 and Videoclip 56.1).

Hospital Course

Surgery was successfully performed. Operative exploration revealed that the tumor was a hemorrhagic, ovoid, soft mass, covered by glistening endocardium (membrane), arose from the interventricular septum, and extended to the apex of RV (6 cm × 6 cm × 5 cm). Its margin was clear, but stalk was unclear.
Pathological diagnosis was hemangioma.

Practical Handbook of Echocardiography 1st edition. Edited by Jing Ping Sun, Joel Felner and John Merlino. © 2010 Blackwell Publishing Ltd.

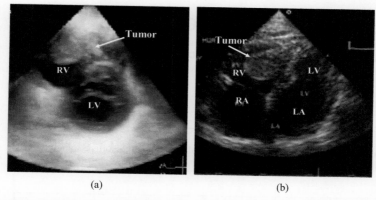

(a)   (b)

Figure 56.1. Transthoracic echocardiography: parasternal short-axis view shows a 60 × 40 mm² mass in the right ventricular outflow tract (a). This mass has a clear boundary and a stalk attached to anteroseptal lower part (b). LA, left atrium; LV, left ventricle; RA, right atrium; RV, right ventricle.

Discussion

The incidence of hemangiomas is 0.8–5% of all benign primary cardiac tumors [1].

Symptoms depend on location and size of the tumor. RV tumors often present with right heart failure as a result of obstruction to RV filling or outflow [1]. Clinical presentations can include shortness of breath, palpitations, atypical chest pain, fatigue, peripheral edema, hepatomegaly, and ascites.

Cardiac tumors have been diagnosed by echocardiography, computed tomography, and magnetic resonance imaging. Bizzard *et al.* found that 21% of cardiac hemangiomas involved the anterior wall of RV, 21% the lateral wall of left ventricle (LV) and 17% the interventricular septum [1]. Studies indicated that the location of hemangiomas in order of frequency were RV, LV, atrial septum, and right atrium [2].

The prognosis for a resectable cardiac hemangioma is usually good, in contrast to unresectable cases which have a poor prognosis and may lead to ventricular arrhythmia, local progression and sudden death. However, recently late recurrence of a cardiac hemangioma has been reported [3]. Therefore, careful follow-up of hemangiomas is required to detect the recurrence of tumor.

References

1. Brizard C, Latremouille C, Jebara VA, *et al.* Cardiac hemangiomas. *Ann Thorac Surg* 1993;56:390–94.
2. Fukusawa S, Yamamoto T, Shimada K. Hemangioma of left ventricular cavity presumptive diagnosis by MRI. *Heart Vessels* 1993;8:211–14.
3. Colli A, Budillon AM, DeCicco G, *et al.* Recurrence of a right ventricular hemangioma. *Thorac Cardiovasc Surg* 2003;126:881–3.

57 Pheochromocytoma

Jing Ping Sun, Angela K. Sullivan, Dan Sorescu & John D. Merlino
Emory University School of Medicine; Emory University Hospital Midtown, Atlanta, GA, USA

History

A 60-year old male admitted because of a syncopal episode associated with unstable blood pressure (BP).

Physical Examination

Heart was in regular sinus rhythm. No murmurs or gallops heard. There were severe fluctuations of BP ranging from systolic blood pressure (SBP) of 60–200 mmHg.

Laboratory

Cardiac catheterization: There was no evidence of significant coronary artery disease.

Severe fluctuations of BP ranging from SBP 60–200 mmHg occurred during the procedure. An intra-aortic balloon pump was placed for hemodynamic support.

Echocardiography: left ventricle (LV) size and systolic function were normal. There was mild left ventricular hypertrophy. The left ventricular outflow tract velocity was normal (1.20 m/sec). During the study, patient developed nonsustained ventricular tachycardia and his LV ejection fraction dropped to <20 with segmental wall motion abnormalities (Videoclips 57.1 and 57.2). The ejection fraction range extended from 5 to 65%.

Computed tomography scan of the abdomen: The presence of a large right adrenal mass (10.3 cm) was identified.

Hospital Course

The patient was placed on alpha blockers. His hypertension was controlled with labetalol. His vascular space was repleted with intravenously administered saline.

Plasma and urinary catecholamines and their metabolic products were grossly abnormal. After control of his hypertension, he was taken to surgery and underwent a right adrenalectomy. He was discharged home on no antihypertensive medications.

Discussion

Pheochromocytoma is a neuroendocrine tumor of the adrenal medulla (originating in the chromaffin cells) or extra-adrenal chromaffin tissue which failed to involute after birth [1]. It secretes excessive amounts of catecholamines, usually epinephrine and norepinephrine. The symptoms and severity of hypertension associated with pheochromocytoma are highly variable, depending on the secretory pattern and amount of catecholamines released. With tumors that continuously release catecholamines, there may be either sustained hypertension with few paroxysms, or sudden bursts of very high BP levels. Tumors that are less active may have cyclical release of catecholamines that induce paroxysms of hypertension.

The clinical presentation also depends on whether the predominant catecholamine that is secreted is norepinephrine or epinephrine. Norepinephrine produces α-adrenergically mediated vasoconstriction with diastolic hypertension, whereas epinephrine produces β-adrenergically mediated cardiac stimulation with mainly systolic hypertension, and tachycardia, associated with sweating, tremors, and flushing. Patients with predominantly epinephrine-secreting tumors sometimes have hypertension alternating with hypotension.

Pheochromocytoma is a rare entity. It is important to record the BP during episodes of apparent anxiety.

The differential diagnosis of pheochromocytoma is Tako-tsubo syndrome. It is characterized by transient wall-motion in the absence of obstructive epicardial coronary disease. One of its mechanisms is catecholamine hypersecretion. Pheochromocytoma may induce myocardial infarction during hypertensive crisis. Though there are similarities with our case, these lesions are distinct clinical entities. The link between these two conditions is catecholamine-induced cardiac-toxicity.

Reference

1. Boulpaep EL, Boron WF. *Medical Physiology: A Cellular and Molecular Approach*. Philadelphia: Saunders, 2003. p. 1065.

58 Left Atrial Mass Caused by Lung Cancer

Ming-Jui Hung

Chang Gung University College of Medicine; Chang Gung Memorial Hospital at Keelung, Keelung, Taiwan.

History

A 60-year old male recently presented with malaise and increasing shortness of breath.

Physical Examination

He appeared to be chronically ill. Blood pressure was 125/78 mmHg, heart rate was 105 bpm with regular rhythm, respiratory rate was 20 and temperature 36.7°C.

Decreased breath sounds and dullness to percussion were found on right lung. Heart sounds were normal. Abdomen was distended with shifting dullness.

Laboratory

Chest X-ray revealed right upper lung mass and right pleural effusions confirmed by computed tomography (CT). A mass was found in left atrium (LA) by transthoracic echocardiography (Figure 58.1 and Videoclip 58.1). A portion of LA mass floated into left ventricle (LV) during diastole. The LV ejection fraction is 66% without significant valvular dysfunction or pericardial involvement. CT-guided biopsy of the mass showed squamous cell carcinoma. A diagnosis of squamous cell lung cancer stage IV was made.

Management

He received supportive care initially; however, he developed ischemic stroke 1 week after admission. The brain CT showed right frontal lobe infarction, which was suggested due to dislodged LA mass. The patient refused operation for his LA mass and his general condition remained unchanged.

Practical Handbook of Echocardiography 1st edition. Edited by Jing Ping Sun, Joel Felner and John Merlino. © 2010 Blackwell Publishing Ltd.

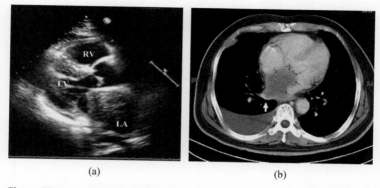

(a)   (b)

Figure 58.1. Parasternal long-axis view shows a mass in the left atrium (arrow, (a)). Computed tomography -contrast enhanced image of right lung mass directly from the right pulmonary vein (arrow) into the left atrium (arrow) (b). LA, left atrium; LV, left ventricle; RV, right ventricle.

Discussion

Metastatic tumors of the heart are far more common than primary cardiac tumors [1]. Many tumor types, such as breast and lung cancer, lymphoma, melanoma, and various sarcomas, have been reported to metastasize to the heart [2]. Lung cancer is the most commonly encountered metastatic tumor at autopsy; however, melanoma has the highest frequency of metastasis to the heart [3]. The development of tachycardia, arrhythmias, cardiomegaly, or heart failure in a patient with carcinoma raises the possibility of cardiac metastasis. Rarely, pericardial effusion or cardiac tamponade is the first manifestation of cardiac involvement by malignant tumors [4].

Lung and breast cancer tend to invade parietal pericardium and then pericardium leading to myocardial constriction and/or pericardial effusion. Isolated or multiple LV neoplastic deposits also are not uncommon [5]. In the setting of cardiac metastatic cancer, all management is palliative. Choice of treatment depends on the primary tumors.

Our case demonstrated that echocardiography is a useful tool to evaluate and predict the dynamic process of intra-cardiac mass. It further emphasized the importance of always performing a complete echocardiogram, including multiple views, and carefully analyzing all available images. This is crucial in patients who may have sequelae secondary to the intra-cardiac mass.

References

1. Abraham KP, Reddy V, Gattuso P. Neoplasms metastatic to the heart: review of 3314 consecutive autopsies. *Am J Cardiovasc Pathol* 1990;3:195–8.
2. Neragi-Miandoab S, Kim J, Vlahakes GJ. Malignant tumours of the heart: a review of tumour type, diagnosis and therapy. *Clin Oncol (R Coll Radiol)* 2007;19:748–56.

3. Mukai K, Shinkai T, Tominaga K, Shimosato Y. The incidence of secondary tumors of the heart and pericardium: a 10-year study. *Jpn J Clin Oncol* 1988;18:195–201.
4. Shapiro LM. Cardiac tumours: diagnosis and management. *Heart* 2001;85:218–22.
5. Roberts WC. Primary and secondary neoplasms of the heart. *Am J Cardiol* 1997;80:671–82.

59 Cardiac Rhabdomyomas

Jing Ping Sun[1], Xing Sheng Yang[1] & James D. Thomas[2]

[1]Emory University School of Medicine; Emory University Hospital Midtown, Atlanta, GA, USA
[2]The Cleveland Clinic Foundation, Cleveland, OH, USA

History and Examination

Case 1. An 8-year old boy with a history of seizures. Examination of the cardiovascular system revealed normal heart sounds and a grade 3/6 ejection systolic murmur in the left upper parasternal region, conducted widely to all areas of the precordium and back.

Case 2. A 3-year old boy presenting congestive heart failure admitted to the hospital. There was no history or clinical signs of tuberous sclerosis in his family.

Laboratory

In case 1, chest X-ray and electrocardiogram were normal.

Echocardiography revealed (1) parasternal long-axis (PLA) view with multiple rhabdomyoma; two tumors are visible in left ventricle (LV), one at the apex and another one at posterior wall. A third tumor is present in left ventricular outflow tract (LVOT). The fourth one is in the right ventricular outflow tract (RVOT), just below the pulmonic valve (Figure 59.1, Videoclip 59.1a).

In case 2, PLA views with two rhabdomyoma: One tumor is in RV, another one is visible in LVOT (a), and almost block the aortic root (Figure 59.2). There is another mass in RV, which can be well seen in Videoclip 59.1b.

Discussion

Cardiac rhabdomyoma is the most common benign cardiac tumor. The tumor is found in more than 50% of children with tuberous sclerosis complex [1]. These cardiac tumors can be partial or complete resolution or to increase/decrease in size with age in some patients [2]. Although any cardiac chamber may be affected, LV is the most frequently involved site [3].

The incidence of symptomatic rhabdomyomas in infancy in the UK has been estimated to be 1 in 326,000 [2].

Cardiac rhabdomyoma is frequently multiple and asymptomatic, but may cause heart failure by causing outflow obstruction, arrhythmias, and

Practical Handbook of Echocardiography 1st edition. Edited by Jing Ping Sun,
Joel Felner and John Merlino. © 2010 Blackwell Publishing Ltd.

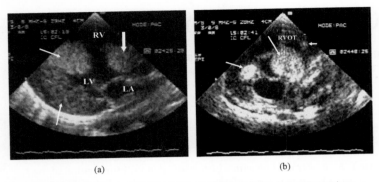

(a)   (b)

Figure 59.1. PLA view (case 1) with multiple rhabdomyoma. Two tumors (arrows) are visible in LV: one at posterior wall, another one (arrow) is present in LVOT (A). Parasternal short axis view shows the third one (small arrow) is in RVOT just below the pulmonic valve (B). LA, left atrium; LV, left ventricle; RV, right ventricle; RVOT, right ventricular outflow tract.

thromboembolic disease. There were four cardiac rhabdomyomas in case 1, one tumor was in the left ventricular outflow tract (LVOT), which may cause seizure; one tumor was located in the RVOT and obstructed it, which lead to heart failure in case 2.

Diagnosis depends on a high index of suspicion and can almost always be made by echocardiography. Both transthoracic echocardiogram and transesophageal echocardiogram images can demonstrate a tumor and its relation to the cardiac chambers and septum as our cases.

The prognosis depends on the site, size, and number of tumors. The presence of cardiac arrhythmias or nonimmune hydrops indicates a poor prognosis. Spontaneous tumor resolution is common, and treatment is therefore usually conservative. The patient is usually followed clinically unless the tumor gives rise to LVOT obstruction, left ventricular failure, or arrhythmias.

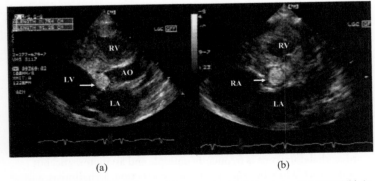

(a)   (b)

Figure 59.2. PLA views with two rhabdomyoma in case 2. One tumor (arrow) is visible in LVOT (A). Parasternal short axis view shows the mass almost block the aortic root (B). AO, aorta; LA, left atrium; LV, left ventricle; RA, right atrium; RV, right ventricle.

References

1. Harding CO, Pagon RA. Incidence of tuberous sclerosis in patients with cardiac rhabdomyoma. *Am J Med Genet* 1990;37:443–6.
2. Freedom RM, Lee KJ, MacDonald C, Taylor G. Selected aspects of cardiac tumors in infancy and childhood. *Pediatr Cardiol* 2000;21:299–316.
3. Black MD, Kadletz M, Smallhorn JF, Freedom RM. Cardiac rhabdomyomas and obstructive left heart disease: histologically but not functionally benign. *Ann Thorac Surg* 1998;65:1388–90.

60 Cardiac Myxomas

Jing Ping Sun[1], Xing Sheng Yang[1], Hong Tang[2] & Joel M. Felner[3]
[1] Emory University School of Medicine; Emory University Hospital Midtown, Atlanta, GA, USA
[2] Sichuan University, Chengdu, Sichuan, China
[3] Grady Memorial Hospital; Emory University School of Medicine, Atlanta, GA, USA

Myxomas account for 40–50% of primary cardiac tumors. Approximately 90% are solitary and pedunculated. Cardiac myxomas are most common in adults, accounting for nearly half of primary cardiac tumors [1]. They are relatively rare in infants and children. Sporadic myxomas occur with a greater frequency among middle-aged women. A left atrium (LA) myxoma was first described in 1845. Most intracardiac myxomas are located in both LA and right atrium (RA) (75–85%), RA (18–25%), right ventricle (RV) (4%), and left ventricle (3%). Approximately 5% of myxoma patients show a familial pattern of tumor development based on autosomal dominant inheritance; 20% of those with myxoma have an abnormal DNA genotype chromosomal pattern [2].

Clinical Presentation

The symptoms and cardiac signs depend on the size, mobility, and location of tumors. Although asymptomatic patients with myxoma have been reported, most present with one or more effects of a triad of constitutional, embolic, and obstructive manifestations. Cardiac myxomas provoke systemic manifestations in 90% of the patients, characterized by weight loss, fatigue, fever, anemia, elevated sedimentation rate, and elevated serum immunoglobulin concentration formed in response to tumor embolization and degenerative changes within the tumor.

Episodes of syncope or dizziness are frequent. Sudden death may occur in 15% of patients with atrial myxoma. Death is typically caused by coronary or systemic embolization or by obstruction of blood flow at the mitral or tricuspid valve.

Laboratory

The value of transthoracic echocardiography (TTE) in the noninvasive diagnosis of intracavitary tumors is well documented. M-mode recording was the primary noninvasive technique for the diagnosis of cardiac

Practical Handbook of Echocardiography 1st edition. Edited by Jing Ping Sun, Joel Felner and John Merlino. © 2010 Blackwell Publishing Ltd.

myxoma for nearly two decades. Figure 60.1 showed M-mode recording of RV and TV in a patient with RA myxoma. The tumor echoes appear in the tricuspid valvular orifice approximately 40 msec post TV opening and fill the region behind the valve for the remaining diastolic period (a). The gross appearance of myxoma (b).

Two-D echocardiography has improved the sensitivity and specificity in the diagnosis of cardiac myxomas. TTE and transesophageal echocardiography can identify the size, shape, location, point of attachment, and motion characteristics of cardiac myxomas. Doppler assessment of the flow patterns provides further information regarding the hemodynamic consequences of myxomas. Atrial myxomas are characteristically rounded or ovoid echogenic masses that are mobile and have cystic changes in some cases.

Three-dimensional echocardiography can show a three dimensional image of the tumor.

The different sizes, locations of myxomas are shown (Figures 60.2 and 60.3, Videoclips 60.1 and 60.2).

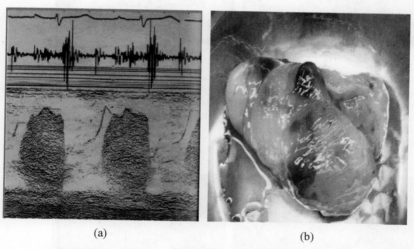

(a)   (b)

Figure 60.1. M-mode recording of right ventricle and tricuspid valve in a patient with right atrial myxoma. The tumor echoes appear in the tricuspid valvular orifice approximately 40 msec post tricuspid valve opening and fill the region behind the valve for the remaining diastolic period (a). The gross appearance of myxoma (b).

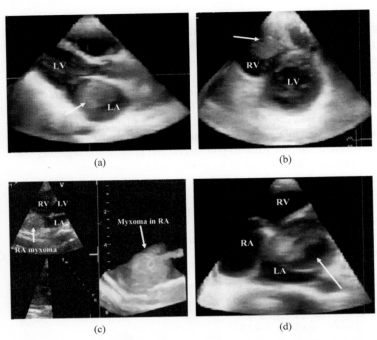

Figure 60.2. Parasternal views from a patient with a left atrial myxoma. Parasternal long axis view shows the tumor originates from the interatrial septum (arrow, a). Parasternal short-axis view shows a myxoma in the right ventricular outflow tract (arrow, b). An apical 4-chamber view demonstrates a mass in the right atrium ((c), left) and the three-dimensional image shows the shape of the tumor (c, right). An left atrial cystic mass is seen in the apical 4-chamber view (d). LA, left atrium; LV, left ventricle; RA, right atrium; RV, right ventricle.

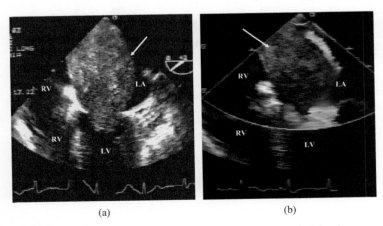

Figure 60.3. Transesophageal echocardiography: A huge myxoma in the left atrium obstructs mitral inflow (a). Color Doppler demonstrates high-velocity flow around the mass and into right ventricle (b). LA, left atrium; LV, left ventricle; RV, right ventricle.

Treatment

Surgical resection of a myxoma is the only acceptable therapy and, in view of the dangers of embolization and sudden death, should be performed as soon as possible, the long-term prognosis is excellent, and recurrences are rare [1].

Reference

1. Reeder GS, Khandheria BK, Seward JB, *et al.* Transesophageal echocardiography and cardiac masses. *Mayo Clin Proc* 1991;66:1101–9.
2. Reynen K. Cardiac myxomas. *N Engl J Med* 1995;333:1610–17.

61 Carcinoid Heart Disease

Jing Ping Sun, Xing Sheng Yang, Alicia N. Rangosch & John D. Merlino
Emory University School of Medicine; Emory University Hospital Midtown, Atlanta, GA, USA

History

A 50-year old complains of tachycardia, and shortness of breath for a month.

Physical Examination

Exam remarkable for hypotension, tachycardia, anasarca, and jugular venous distension. Systolic murmurs were heard at both the base of the heart and the left lower sternal border.

Laboratory

Transthoracic echocardiography revealed right ventricle (RV) and right atrium (RA) dilation; tricuspid valve (TV) leaflets were thickened in appearance, and reduced mobility with severe tricuspid regurgitation (TR) and stenosis (Figures 61.1 and 61.2, Videoclip 61.1). The mean gradient by Doppler across the TV was 5.9 mmHg.

The pulmonic valve was thickened with mild pulmonic regurgitation. (Videoclip 61.2). The estimated gradient of pulmonary artery was 54 mmHg.

Discussion

Cardiac involvement has been recognized in more than 50% of patients with carcinoid tumors. These patients develop extensive fibrous deposits on the endocardial interfaces of the right side of the heart [1]. These deposits interfere with normal myocardial and valvular function; as a result, heart failure is the leading cause of death.

Practical Handbook of Echocardiography 1st edition. Edited by Jing Ping Sun, Joel Felner and John Merlino. © 2010 Blackwell Publishing Ltd.

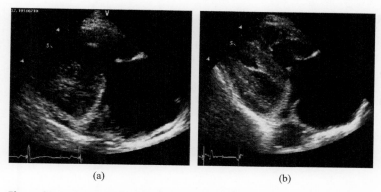

(a)   (b)

Figure 61.1. The tricuspid valves are thickened and fixed, the leaflets cannot open widely during diastole (a), and cannot close tightly during systole (b).

The predilection for right-sided valve disease in carcinoid syndrome is most likely related to the serotonin-rich blood that enters the right atrium directly from the liver and the subsequent partial pulmonary degradation of serotonin [2]. In rare cases, the tumor involves left-sided heart valves and myocardium [3]. The diagnosis of carcinoid heart disease is difficult, and as in our patient, the diagnosis is often not made until the late in the disease. Heart murmurs and the symptom of dyspnea are noted more frequently among patients with carcinoid heart disease versus those without [3]. TR is present in all patients.

Normally, the hepatic vein drains into inferior vena cava and right atrium during systole in response to the fall in the atrial pressure. In patient with severe tricuspid regurgitation, because of RV contraction causes sustained retrograde flow through RA back up into inferior vena cava system indicated by systolic flow reversal in the hepatic vein. These are typical signs for severe tricuspid regurgitation, which are well demonstrated in our case.

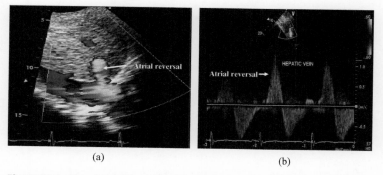

(a)   (b)

Figure 61.2. The subcostal view with color Doppler shows the blood flow is reversed into the hepatic vein during the systolic period of ventricles (a); the Doppler recording is consistent with the color flow (b). These are typical signs of severe tricuspid regurgitation.

References

1. Robiolio PA, Rigolin VH, Wilson JS, *et al.* Carcinoid heart disease: correlation of high serotonin levels with valvular abnormalities detected by cardiac catheterization and echocardiography. *Circulation* 1995;92:790–95.
2. Connolly HM, Crary JL, McGoon MD. Valvular heart disease associated with fenfluramine–phentermine. *N Engl J Med* 1997;337:581–8.
3. Pelliffa PA, Tajik AJ, Khandheria BK, *et al.* Carcinoid heart disease: clinical and echocardiographic spectrum in 74 patients. *Circulation* 1993;87:1188–96.

62 Cardiac Papillary Fibroelastoma

Jing Ping Sun[1], Xing Sheng Yang[1], William J. Stewart[2] & James D. Thomas[2]

[1] Emory University School of Medicine; Emory University Hospital Midtown, Atlanta, GA, USA
[2] The Cleveland Clinic Foundation, Cleveland, OH, USA

Cardiac papillary fibroelastoma (CPF) is a rare primary cardiac neoplasm of unknown prevalence [1]. Since the introduction of echocardiography, the diagnosis of these tumors in living patients has been reported sporadically.

Studied Cases

A total of 162 patients with pathologically proven CPF were identified through the pathology database at the Cleveland Clinic Foundation between March 1, 1983 and March 31, 1999. Patients ranged in age from 5 to 86 years, and 46.1% were male. In this group, 93 patients with 110 CPFs were identified by echocardiography. A total of 48 patients had CPFs confirmed by pathological examination that were not visible on echocardiograms because these CPFs were extremely small (<0.2 cm).

On the echocardiographic studies, tumors appeared round, oval, or irregular, but were generally well-demarcated and homogenous in appearance. When image quality was optimal, a "speckled appearance" with "stippling" around the perimeter could be seen [2]. Among the 110 CPFs seen by echocardiography, 49 (44.5%) were on the aortic cusp (24 on the right, 6 on the left, and 19 on the noncoronary cusp), with 40 tumors present on the aortic side of the valve (Figure 62.1a, Videoclip 62.1) and 9 on the ventricular side. Forty tumors (36.4%) were on the mitral leaflets (23 on the anterior and 17 on the posterior leaflet) (Figure 62.2b, Videoclip 62.1), with 32 in the left atrium (Figure 62.1c and 62.1c) and 8 in the left ventricle. Significantly more tumors occurred on the valves than in chambers (91 of 110, 82.7%, versus 19 of 110, 17.3%; $P < 0.001$). The size of the tumors ranged from 2 to 28 mm for the largest dimension. A total of 99% were <20 mm. Comparison of tumor size measured by pathology and echocardiography in a subgroup of 45 patients shows a good correlation between two methods (Figure 62.2).

The masses in the cardiac chambers were larger than those on the aortic or mitral valves (12.0 ± 4.6 mm versus 8.5 ± 4.4 mm in diameter, respectively; $P < 0.001$). All 19 CPFs in the chambers were mobile, as were 29 of the 91 on a valvular surface (31.9%). Single lesions were detected by echocardiography in 85 patients (91.4%). Multiple CPFs (range, 2–8) were

Practical Handbook of Echocardiography 1st edition. Edited by Jing Ping Sun, Joel Felner and John Merlino. © 2010 Blackwell Publishing Ltd.

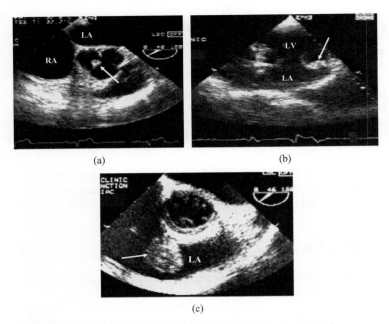

Figure 62.1. Transesophageal echocardiography short-axis view shows a small fibroelastoma on the aortic noncoronary (a). An apical 4-chamber view shows a fibroelastoma on the mitral posterior leaflet (b). Transesophageal echocardiography short-axis view shows a fibroelastoma in the left atrium (c). LA, left atrium; LV, left ventricle; RA, right atrium. Reproduced with permission from Elsevier.

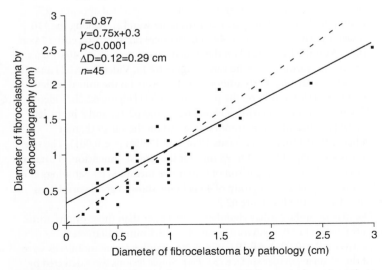

Figure 62.2. Comparison of tumor size measured by pathology and echocardiography in a subgroup of 45 patients shows a good correlation between two methods. Reproduced with permission from Elsevier.

detected in eight patients (8.6%). One patient had eight tumors observed in various locations on the right and left sides of the heart.

Echocardiographic follow-up data was available for 64 of 141 patients (45.4%) after surgical excision. The average follow-up time was 630 ± 903 days. No mass was detected by echocardiography in any patient during the follow-up period.

Discussion

We found that the typical echocardiographic features of CPF included (1) the tumor is round, oval, or irregular in appearance, with well-demarcated borders and a homogeneous texture; (2) most CPFs are small (99% were <20 mm in the largest dimension); (3) nearly half of CPFs had small stalks, and those with stalks were mobile; (4) CPFs may be single or multiple lesions and are most often associated with cardiac valvular disease. Approximately 90% of the CPFs reported in the literature were attached to valves [3], and the majority were on the aortic valve [3]. In our group, 49 of the 110 CPFs (44.5%) were attached to the aortic valve, predominantly on the aortic side. The mitral valve was the next most common location [1].

Our study found that CPFs were usually <20 mm in their largest diameter; stalks and mobility were present in most patients. As expected, these traits may be associated with the likelihood of embolization. There were eight CPFs on both sides of the heart in one patient of our group. In our study, CPFs were diagnosed incidentally in many patients with another underlying cardiovascular disease who were asymptomatic.

Echocardiography is a convenient and noninvasive diagnostic technique and should be the first choice of tests to search for CPFs. Transesophageal echocardiography is an important tool for delineating the extent and anatomic attachment of these small tumors.

The reasons echocardiography may fail to diagnose tumors include (1) the tumor was masked by an associated lesion; (2) the tumor was too small to be seen; (3) the examination was not done carefully with a sufficient index of suspicion; or (4) there were no significant characteristics to differentiate the CPF from the degenerative valve disease. Decisions regarding the primary surgical excision of CPF depend on the size, location, mobility, and potential or strength of association of the tumor with symptoms.

References

1. Burke A, Virmani R. Tumors of the heart and great vessels. In: *Atlas of Tumor Pathology*, Third Series. Washington DC: Armed Forces Institute of Pathology, 1996, pp. 47–54.
2. Israel DH, Sherman W, Ambrose JA, *et al*. Dynamic coronary ostial obstruction due to papillary fibroelastoma leading to myocardial ischemia and infarction. *Am J Cardiol* 1991;67:104–5.
3. McAllister HA, Jr, Fengolio JJ, Jr. Papillary fibroelastoma. In: Landing BH (eds) *Tumors of the Cardiovascular System*. Washington DC: Armed Forces Institute of Pathology, 1978, pp. 20–25.

63 Cardiac Fibroma

Jing Ping Sun[1] & James D. Thomas[2]

[1] Emory University School of Medicine; Emory University Hospital Midtown, Atlanta, GA, USA
[2] The Cleveland Clinic Foundation, Cleveland, OH, USA

History

An 18-year-old male with elevated blood pressure on physical for baseball.

Physical Examination

Unremarkable except for elevated blood pressure (168/96 mmHg).

Laboratory

Stress test: small regions of peri-infarct ischemia in left coronary territory were found.

Echocardiogram: a mass at the left ventricle (LV) apex with small pericardial effusion was found (Figure 63.1).

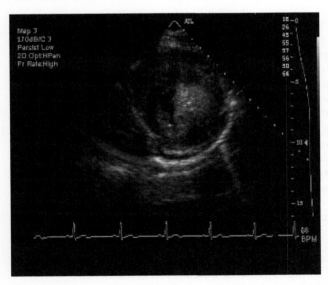

Figure 63.1. Parasternal short-axis view shows a tumor in myocardium of left ventricular lateral wall.

Practical Handbook of Echocardiography 1st edition. Edited by Jing Ping Sun, Joel Felner and John Merlino. © 2010 Blackwell Publishing Ltd.

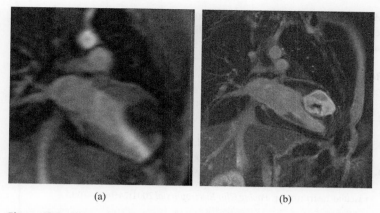

(a)   (b)

Figure 63.2. The magnetic resonance images showed a regular mass in the myocardium of the lateral free wall of the left ventricle close to the apex (a). Magnetic resonance images postgadolinium enhancement (b).

The magnetic resonance images showed a regular mass in the myocardium of LV lateral wall close to the apex (Figure 63.2).

Treatment

The patient was referred to cardiothoracic surgery for complete resection of a benign neoplasm. After operation, he resumed normal sports activities.

Surgical/pathologic findings: Cardiac fibroma measuring 8 cm × 6 cm × 6 cm was found. It was completely encapsulated and was with irregular margins.

Discussion

Cardiac fibromas are considered low-grade connective tissue tumors derived from fibroblasts. This has been well-documented with serial echocardiograms and magnetic resonance imaging. The vast majority of fibromas are found either within the LV free wall or within the interventricular septum. Approximately 70% of these lesions become symptomatic at some point [1]. Most commonly, they cause flow obstruction or conduction disturbances. The most prevalent arrhythmia is ventricular tachycardia or fibrillation. The incidence of sudden death is estimated to be 30% [2].

When patients become symptomatic, surgical excision usually leads to a favorable outcome [3]. However, when lesions are unresectable, other solutions should be sought. A review of the literature reveals three cases where unresectable benign tumors causing malignant arrhythmias were managed with the insertion of an implantable cardioverter defibrillator [4]. However, no postimplantation follow-up was reported in those studies.

Malignant arrhythmias secondary to an unresectable cardiac fibroma may require transplantation. The main indication for transplantation has been cardiac inflow or outflow obstruction that resulted in cardiac failure.

References

1. Beghetti M, Gow RM, Haney I, *et al.* Pediatric primary benign cardiac tumors: a 15-year review. *Am Heart J* 1997;134:1107–14.
2. Kusano KF, Ohe T. Cardiac tumors that cause arrhythmias. *Card Electrophysiol Rev* 2002;6:174–7.
3. Yamaguchi M, Hosokawa Y, Ohashi H, *et al.* Cardiac fibroma: long term fate after excision. *J Thorac Cardiovasc Surg* 1992;103:140.
4. Thogersen AM, Helvind M, Jensen T, *et al.* Implantable cardioverter defibrillator in a 4-month-old infant with cardiac arrest associated with a vascular heart tumor. *Pacing Clin Electrophysiol* 2001;24:1699–700.

64 Right-Sided Cardiac Metastatic Pleomorphic Sarcoma

Jing Ping Sun[1] & James D. Thomas[2]

[1] Emory University School of Medicine; Emory University Hospital Midtown, Atlanta, GA, USA
[2] The Cleveland Clinic Foundation, Cleveland, OH, USA

History

A 50-year old man presented with a history of sarcoma in buttock 1 year post operation.

Physical Examination

A grade 2/6 systolic murmur is heard throughout the precordium.

Echocardiography

A 42 × 46 mm^2 immobile mass was noted in the right ventricle (RV), which was fixed to the apical and mid free wall as well as the apical septum (Figure 64.1, Videoclip 64.1) The RV was dilated.

The right atrium (RA) was moderately dilated. The interatrial septum bowed toward the left during atrial contraction consistent with elevated RA pressure. LV was normal in size and systolic function, the septum bowed toward LV during systole suggesting right sided pressure overload (Videoclip 64.2).

Magnetic resonance imaging revealed a mass in RV. The mass was heterogeneous in signal on steady-state-free-precession imaging, isointense on a fast high-resolution multislice T1-weighted turbo spin-echo (TSE) imaging, and hyperintense on T2 TSE imaging.

Pathology

The buttock mass is examined by pathology and diagnosed as a high-grade pleomorphic undifferentiated sarcoma with myxoid.

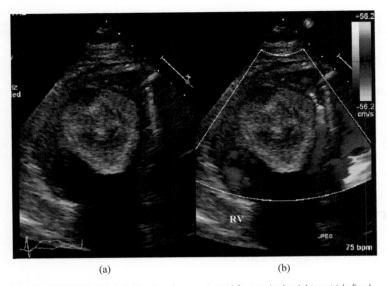

(a)　　　　　　　　　　　(b)

Figure 64.1. Apical 4-chamber view shows an immobile mass in the right ventricle fixed to the apical and mid free wall (a). Color flow around the tumor can be seen (b). RV, right ventricle.

Discussion

Soft-tissue sarcomas are rare causes of metastatic tumors of the heart, which often involve the right side of the heart and rarely present as intracavitary lesions [1]. Metastatic heart tumors occur more frequently at a rate that is at least 100 times higher than that of primary tumors, and typically in patients with disseminated disease [2]. Myxoid liposarcomas, which have a tendency to metastasize to extrapulmonary tissues without pulmonary involvement, represent the most common extremity sarcoma to metastasize to the heart [3]. Cardiac metastasis from an undifferentiated pleomorphic sarcoma is uncommon [4]. Cardiac metastatic tumors generally infiltrate the myocardium and pericardium and rarely involve the endocardium or the valves [1].

Two-dimensional echocardiography is the diagnostic method of choice, and TEE approach can confirm anatomical location, quantify baseline valvular dysfunction, and guide cannulation and transvenous biopsy before the administration of chemotherapy [1]. Apart from tumor, the differential diagnosis of an intracardiac mass should include thrombus, vegetation, and a foreign body. The treatment for cardiac sarcoma depends largely upon the location and size of the tumor, as well as the extent of metastasis.

References
1. Reynen K, Kockeritz U, Strasser RH. Metastases to the heart. *Ann Oncol* 2004;15:375–81.

2. Butany J, Nair V, Naseemuddin A, *et al.* Cardiac tumours: diagnosis and management. *Lancet Oncol* 2005;6:219–28.
3. Estourgie SH, Nielsen GP, Ott MJ. Metastatic patterns of extremity myxoid liposarcoma and their outcome. *J Surg Oncol* 2002;80:89–93.
4. Burke AP, Cowan D, Virmani R. Primary sarcomas of the heart. *Cancer* 1992;69:387–95.

65 Primary Cardiac Undifferentiated Sarcoma

Jing Ping Sun[1], Xing Sheng Yang[1] & James D. Thomas[2]

[1] Emory University School of Medicine; Emory University Hospital Midtown, Atlanta, GA, USA
[2] The Cleveland Clinic Foundation, Cleveland, OH, USA

History

A 30-year-old female complains of chest pain and rapidly progressive dyspnea.

Physical Examination

Blood pressure was 110/70 mmHg; pulse was regular (135/minute), and respiration rate was 24/minute. Cardiac auscultation revealed a grade 3/6 systolic murmur at the precordial area.

Laboratory

Electrocardiogram showed sinus tachycardia. Chest X-ray revealed bilateral pulmonary edema.

Echocardiography: parasternal long-axis view showed a large mass on basal segment of interventricular septum. The mass was identified as undifferentiated sarcoma by pathology. The tumor partially obstructed left ventricular outflow tract (LVOT) (Figure 65.1 and Videoclip 65.1).

Discussion

Primary malignant tumors of the heart are rare [1], and almost all are sarcomas. Undifferentiated cardiac sarcomas primarily develop on the left side of the heart and cause signs and symptoms related to pulmonary congestion, mitral stenosis, and pulmonary vein obstruction [2]. The clinical symptoms and signs should be related with the size and location of the tumor. The tumor was on the basal ventricular septum almost obstructing LVOT causing dyspnea and pulmonary edema in our case.

Transthoracic echocardiography is usually the first elective procedure for the diagnosis of cardiac tumors. Transesophageal echocardiography is very useful for a more detailed evaluation [3]. With these techniques, tumors

Practical Handbook of Echocardiography 1st edition. Edited by Jing Ping Sun,
Joel Felner and John Merlino. © 2010 Blackwell Publishing Ltd.

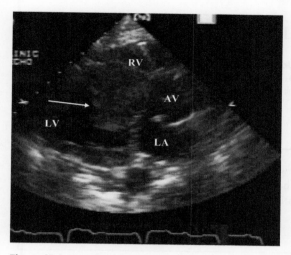

Figure 65.1. Parasternal long-axis view shows a large mass (arrow) located in the interventricular septum. It is identified as undifferentiated sarcoma. It partially obstructs the left ventricular outflow tract. AV, aortic valve; LA, left atrium; LV, left ventricle; RV, right ventricle.

are displayed as masses variable in size and characteristics, such as shape, possible valve involvement, and myocardial invasion of the tumor; therefore, they provide useful information for determining the optimal therapeutic approach.

Surgical treatment usually is much more difficult because the tumor is often so large at the time of diagnosis that complete resection is not possible. When the tumor is limited in size, complete resection with valve reconstruction or replacement when necessary must be undertaken because of survival improvement.

Some studies revealed that adjuvant therapy for cardiac tumors may be only a palliative measure since it does not improve survival [4].

The prognosis of cardiac primary sarcoma is very poor after the first symptoms, because cardiac sarcomas rapidly infiltrate all layers of the heart and further invade adjacent mediastinal structures.

References

1. Reynen K. Frequency of primary tumors of the heart. *Am J Cardiol* 1996;77:107.
2. Allard MF, Taylor GP, Wilson JE, *et al.* Primary cardiac tumors. In: Goldhaber SZ, Braunwald E (eds) *Atlas of Heart Disease*, Vol. 3: *Cardiopulmonary Disease and Cardiac Tumors*. St Louis: Mosby-Year Book, 1995, pp. 1–22.
3. Kulander BG, Polissar L, Yang CY, *et al.* Grading of soft tissue sarcomas: necrosis as a determinant of survival. *Mod Pathol* 1989;2:205–8.
4. Burke AP, Virmani R. *Atlas of Tumor Pathology*, 3rd edition. Washington: Armed Forces Institute of Pathology, 1995.

66 Pericardial Cyst

Jing Ping Sun[1] & Joel M. Felner[2]

[1] Emory University School of Medicine; Emory University Hospital Midtown, Atlanta, GA, USA
[2] Grady Memorial Hospital; Emory University School of Medicine, Atlanta, GA, USA

History

A 40-year-old male was referred to a cardiologist with a symptomatic mass in contact with the heart, which was found by chest X-ray.

Physical examination was normal.

Laboratory

Transthoracic echocardiography: a large pericardial cyst was noted posterolateral to left atrium (LA) from apical 4- and apical 2-chamber views. LA was partially compressed by the cyst. There was no communication between the LA and cyst (Figure 66.1 and Videoclip 66.1).

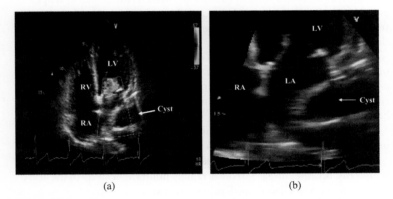

(a) (b)

Figure 66.1. Echocardiogram: apical 4-chamber view indicates that the paracardiac cyst (arrow) is visible as a paracardiac void large sac located laterally to left atrium (a). The area of cyst zoomed in—the pericardial cyst is uniloculus and does not communicate with the pericardial space (b). LA, left atrium; LV, left ventricle; RA, right atrium; RV, right ventricle.

Discussion

Pericardial or mesothelial cysts are the most frequent benign "tumors" of the pericardium. Pericardial cyst is the result of an outpouching of the

Practical Handbook of Echocardiography 1st edition. Edited by Jing Ping Sun, Joel Felner and John Merlino. © 2010 Blackwell Publishing Ltd.

parietal pericardium that is lined by mesothelial cells. Most of the pericardial cysts are uniloculus. They usually contain clear yellow fluid and do not communicate with the pericardial space.

Pericardial cysts occur most frequently in the third or fourth decade of life, equally among men and women.

Generally, pericardial cysts are detected incidentally in asymptomatic patients, as in our case. However, 25–30% of patients will have chest pain, dyspnea, cough, or paroxysmal tachycardia. Only very rarely this is a cause of serious cardiovascular complications, such as acute right-sided heart failure due to hemorrhage into a pericardial cyst [1].

The pericardial cyst may be of almost any size. Rapid change in size, particularly a decrease in size, suggests a pericardial diverticulum rather than a pericardial cyst.

Usually, clinical examination, a plain chest radiograph and echocardiography are sufficient for clinical decision making. In certain cases, however, physicians may prefer to employ more advanced imaging modalities, such as computed tomography, magnetic resonance imaging, which, by its inherent capabilities to characterize tissues and fluids in the human body, may be helpful in the differential diagnosis of thoracic tumors and cysts [2].

In patients with symptoms, various cures are suggested in the literature including open chest surgery [3], puncture of the cyst without or with subsequent ethanol sclerosis or with injection of contrast media, and thoracoscopic resection [2].

The optimal therapeutic approach is dependent on local expertise. Given the low risk inherent to the natural course of even large pericardial cysts, one may favor referral to physicians capable of performing minimally invasive surgical interventions.

References

1. Cangemi V, Volpino P, Gualdi G, *et al.* Pericardial cyst of the mediastinum. *J Cardiovasc Surg* 1999;40:909–13.
2. Eto A, Arima T, Nagashima A. Pericardial cyst in a child treated with video-assisted thoracoscopic surgery. *Eur J Pediatr* 2000;159:889–91.
3. Wychulis AR, Payne WS, Clagett OT. Surgical treatment of mediastinal tumours: a 40 year experience. *J Thorac Cardiovasc Surg* 1971;62:379–91.

67 Left Ventricular Septal Aneurysm in Cardiac Sarcoidosis

Xing Sheng Yang, Jing Ping Sun & John D. Merlino
Emory University School of Medicine; Emory University Hospital Midtown, Atlanta, GA, USA

History

An 80-year-old female was hospitalized with a 1-day history of inability to speak. She had a history of pulmonary and cardiac sarcoidosis, hypertension, and diabetes mellitus.

Laboratory

Electrocardiogram showed atrial fibrillation with rapid ventricular response, ventricular premature beats, and ventricular septal infarct. Brain computed tomography revealed a small focus of low attenuation in the left basal ganglia is most consistent with subacute or chronic lacunar infarction.

Echocardiography

There is mild left ventricular hypertrophy. An apical 4-chamber (A4-ch) view showed thinning of the septal basal and middle segments forming ventricular septal aneurysm (Figure 67.1a and Videoclip 67.1). PLA view showed thinning anteroseptal basal wall (Figure 67.1b). Mild mitral and aortic regurgitation, and severe tricuspid regurgitation (TR). The peak velocity of TR jet is 3 m/sec, with systolic pulmonary pressure of approximately 45 mmHg. The pulmonic valves are normal. A pacemaker is noted in the right ventricle (RV). The RV size and function are normal. The left and right atria are enlarged. There is a minimal pericardial effusion.

Discussion

Sarcoidosis is a multisystem granulomatous disease of unknown origin. Direct myocardial involvement occurs in 13–20% of cases of sarcoidosis. Usually cardiac lesions are local and to scattered and affect mostly the septum and ventricular free wall [1].

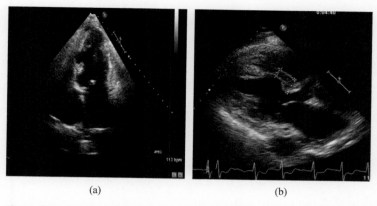

(a)   (b)

Figure 67.1. Apical 4-chamber view shows thinning septal basal and middle segments forming ventriculoseptal aneurysm (a). parasternal long-axis view shows thinning anteroseptal basal wall (b).

Most patients with cardiac sarcoidosis have conduction disturbances or arrhythmias (80%) and /or impaired cardiac function (31%) [2]. It includes valvular involvement, myocardial infarction. Electrocardiogram abnormalities including heart block, other conduction disturbances, arrhythmias, and repolarization abnormalities [3]. The diagnosis of cardiac sarcoidosis is difficult because of the nonspecific nature of the clinical manifestations. The differential diagnosis should include other granulomatous diseases, multiple myocardial abscesses, and myocardial metastases. Historically, thallium scintigraphy, gallium scanning, and echocardiography have been widely used.

Echocardiographic findings have included abnormal septal thickening, pericardial effusion, a focal thin left ventricular wall, and ventricular septal motion abnormalities [4]. Ventricular aneurysms are among the least common manifestations of cardiac sarcoidosis [5]. All characteristics of echocardiographic findings mentioned above are present in our case, as well as pulmonary sarcoidosis.

References

1. Bashour FA, McConnell T, Skinner W, *et al.* Myocardial sarcoidosis. *Dis Chest* 1968;53:413–20.
2. Valantine H, Mckenna WJ, Nihoyannopoutos P, *et al.* Sarcoidosis: a pattern of clinical and morphological presentation. *Br Heart J* 1987;57:256–63.
3. Greif M, Petrakopoulou P, Weiss M, *et al.* Cardiac sarcoidosis concealed by arrhythmogenic right ventricular dysfunction. *Nat Clin Pract Cardiovasc Med* 2008;5:231–6.
4. Chiles C, Adams GW, Ravin CE. Radiographic manifestations of cardiac sarcoidosis. *AJR* 1985;145:711–14.
5. Lewin RF, Mor R, Spitzer S, *et al.* Echocardiographic evaluation of patients with systemic sarcoidosis. *Am Heart J* 1985;110:116–22.

Part 9
Infective Disease

68 Constrictive Pericarditis

Jing Ping Sun[1], Xing Sheng Yang[1] & Joel M. Felner[2]

[1]Emory University School of Medicine; Emory University Hospital Midtown, Atlanta, GA, USA
[2]Grady Memorial Hospital; Emory University School of Medicine, Atlanta, GA, USA

Constrictive pericarditis (CP) is defined as chronic fibrous thickening of the pericardial wall that results in abnormal diastolic filling. CP can be caused by infections, connective-tissue diseases, neoplasms, mechanical trauma, myocardial infarction, amyloid, uremia, open-heart surgery, or mediastinal radiation. The majority of cases appear to be idiopathic or due to occult viral infection. The course of the disease is typically quite slow. Patients with pericardial constriction may present with symptoms suggesting either fluid overload (peripheral edema and anasarca) or diminished cardiac output (easy fatigability and dyspnea on exertion). CP classically causes marked elevation in the jugular venous pressure, hepatomegaly, ascites, and peripheral edema signs that mimic right heart failure. The pericardial thickening, signs of abnormal ventricular filling by M-mode, two-dimensional, and Doppler findings are helpful in diagnosis.

We present several cases with typical echocardiographic signs for reference.

Figure 68.1 and Videoclip 68.1 illustrates: Transthoracic echocardiography and transesophageal echocardiogram (TEE) recordings of four patients with constrictive pericarditis. The thickened and calcified pericardium can be clearly appreciated in subcostal four-chamber view (a). A case with loculated effusion with elements of constriction is shown (b). A purulent pericarditis demonstrated in TEE image (c). The image indicated a case with constrictive pericarditis and pleural effusion (d).

Figure 68.2 shows an M-mode recording of the septal position which varies with respiration, and during inspiration interventricular septum deviates to the left.

Figure 68.3 Doppler and pulse tissue Doppler recordings demonstrated: (a) a marked inspiration fall in peak mitral E-wave velocity (mean >30% from expiration). (b) A large atrial reversal wave (AR) of hepatic vein. Doppler recording indicated high-end diastolic pressure of RV. (c) Peak early longitudinal velocities (E') in patients with constrictive pericarditis are high.

Videoclip 68.2: apical 4-chamber (A4-ch) (a) and parasternal short-axis views (b) show the interventriculoseptal paradoxical motion during respiration.

Practical Handbook of Echocardiography 1st edition. Edited by Jing Ping Sun, Joel Felner and John Merlino. © 2010 Blackwell Publishing Ltd.

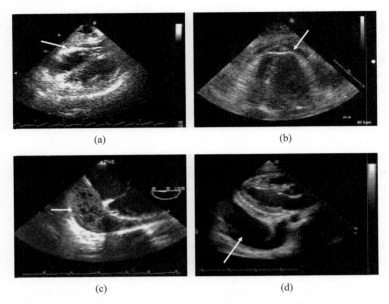

(a)   (b)

(c)   (d)

Figure 68.1. Transthoracic echocardiography and transesophageal echocardiography recordings of four patients with constrictive pericarditis. The thickened and calcified pericardium (arrow) can be clearly appreciated in subcostal four-chamber view (a). A case with loculated effusion with elements of constriction is shown (b). A purulent pericarditis demonstrated in transesophageal echocardiogram image (c). The image indicated a case with constrictive pericarditis and pleural effusion (d).

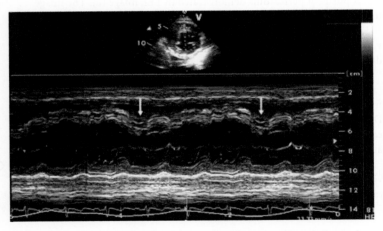

Figure 68.2. M-mode recording shows the septal position varies with respiration, and during inspiration, interventricular septum deviates to the left (arrows).

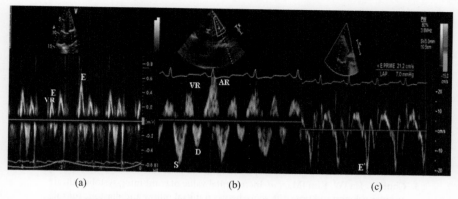

(a)   (b)   (c)

Figure 68.3. Doppler and pulse tissue Doppler recordings demonstrated: (a) a marked inspiratory fall in peak mitral E-wave velocity (mean >30% from expiration). (b) A large atrial reversal wave (AR) of hepatic vein. This Doppler recording indicated the end diastolic pressure of right ventricle is high. (c) Peak early longitudinal velocities (E′) in patients with constrictive pericarditis are high. AR, aortic regurgitation; VR, ventricular reversal.

Discussion

A dissociation between intrathoracic and intracardiac pressures can be detected as reciprocal changes in diastolic flow velocities across the tricuspid and mitral valves during respiration. Doppler signs of constriction are related to the diastolic filling changes in the respiratory phase of both ventricles. Inspiratory decrease of pulmonary wedge pressure subsequently diminished the pulmonic vein–left atrium gradient and therefore delayed mitral valve opening, prolonging isovolumetric relaxation time by approximately 50%. The mitral valve peak E velocity manifested an inspiratory decrease by a mean >30% with a reciprocal increase of peak E velocity of the tricuspid valve by similar values. Inspiration decreased peak systolic aortic flow, slightly increasing the peak pulmonary systolic flow [1]. The inferior vena cava is dilated with lack of inspiratory collapse and hepatic venous flow exhibited a prominent atrial systolic reverse flow, keeping the same relation between forward systolic and diastolic flow waves.

Doppler helps to distinguish between CP and restrictive cardiomyopathy (RCM) by demonstrating respiratory variation in restrictive inflow patterns. Peak early longitudinal axial velocities (E′) in patients with CP are high, but not in RCM. A value of >8.0 cm/sec differentiated patients with CP from those with RCM; the sensitivity and specificity are 89 and 100% respectively [2]. The combination of incremental value of systolic mitral annular velocity (S') and time difference between onset of mitral inflow and onset of E′ (T (E′ − E)) significantly increased sensitivity from 70 to 94% [3]. T (E′ − E) was significantly shorter in patients with CP than with RCM.

The distinction between pericardial constriction and myocardial restriction is very important because CP can improve after pericardiectomy, whereas RCM usually does not.

The treatment of constrictive pericarditis is primarily surgical, but pericardiectomy is difficult to perform late in the course of the disorder. Videoclip 68.2 demonstrates postoperative A4-ch view shows the interventriculoseptal motion returns to normal (a) from its paradoxical motion (b).

References

1. Sun JP, Abdalla IA, Yang XS, *et al.* Respiratory variation of mitral and pulmonary venous Doppler flow velocities in constrictive pericarditis before and after pericardiectomy. *J Am Soc Echocardiogr* 2001;14:1119–26.
2. Rajagopalan N, Garcia MJ, Rodriguez L, *et al.* Comparison of new Doppler echocardiographic methods to differentiate constrictive pericardial heart disease and restrictive cardiomyopathy. *Am J Cardiol* 2001;87:86.
3. Choi EY, Ha JW, Kim JM, *et al.* Incremental value of combining systolic mitral annular velocity and time difference between mitral inflow and diastolic mitral annular velocity to early diastolic annular velocity for differentiating constrictive pericarditis form restrictive cardiomyopathy. *J Am Soc Echocardiogr* 2007;20:738.

69 Aortic Ring Abscess

Jing Ping Sun[1], Xing Sheng Yang[1] & Joel M. Felner[2]

[1]Emory University School of Medicine; Emory University Hospital Midtown, Atlanta, GA, USA
[2]Grady Memorial Hospital; Emory University School of Medicine, Atlanta, GA, USA

History

A 40-year-old man was admitted with fever and marked fatigue.

Physical Examination

Temperature was 40°C; pulse was 124/minute, and respirations were 30/minute. Blood pressure was 130/56 mmHg. A grade 2 systolic murmur was heard at the second rib space and a grade 2 diastolic blowing murmur was heard along the left sternal border.

Laboratory

Chest X-ray radiographs revealed a left-sided pleural effusion and pneumonia in the left lung. Blood cultures were positive for *Staphylococcus aureus*.

Transthoracic echocardiography (TTE): Parasternal views showed mobile vegetations attached to aortic valve leaflets. There was an echo-free space anterior to the aortic root, consistent with an aortic-root abscess. Color Doppler showed moderate-to-severe aortic regurgitation (AR).

Transesophageal echocardiography (TEE): An abscess and vegetation in left ventricular outflow tract attached to the aortic valve were noted (Figure 69.1a). Doppler color-flow mapping revealed severe AR (Figure 69.1b and Videoclip 69.1).

We presented more images from two additional cases with different aortic or septal abscess in Figures 69.2, 69.3 and Videoclip 69.2.

Hospital Course

At surgery, a large aortic-root abscess extending from the left coronary ostia to the origin of right coronary artery, with purulent destruction of part of the interventricular septum were identified. Treatment with intravenous gentamicin and vancomycin began.

Pathology: trileaflet aortic valve with extensive destruction of the noncoronary leaflet, which was covered by a brown, friable vegetation.

Practical Handbook of Echocardiography 1st edition. Edited by Jing Ping Sun, Joel Felner and John Merlino. © 2010 Blackwell Publishing Ltd.

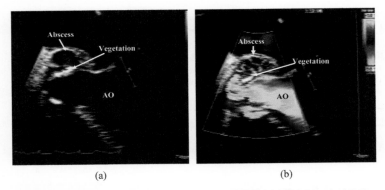

(a)   (b)

Figure 69.1. Transesophageal echocardiography revealed an abscess (small arrow) and a vegetation in left ventricular outflow tract attached to the valve (long arrow) (a), color Doppler shows an aortic abscess (small arrow) and a vegetation in left ventricular outflow tract (long arrow) with severe aortic regurgitation flow (b). AO, aorta.

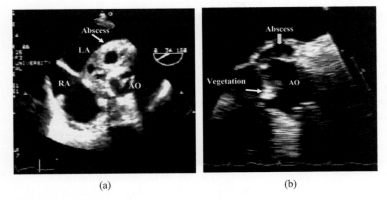

(a)   (b)

Figure 69.2. Transesophageal echocardiography revealed: an abscess (a); an abscess and a vegetation (arrows) (b) in the aortic root. AO, aorta; LA, left atrium; RA, right atrium.

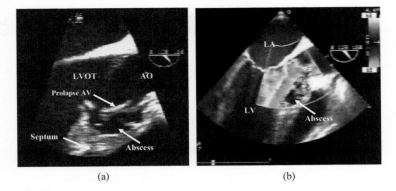

(a)   (b)

Figure 69.3. Transesophageal echocardiography revealed an abscess just below aortic valve; it involved the aortic valve and caused aortic valve prolapse (a), color Doppler shows a broad stream of regurgitant flow due to aortic valve prolapse (b). AO, aorta; AV, aortic valve; LA, left atrium; LV, left ventricle; LVOT, left ventricular outflow tract.

Discussion

Valve ring abscess is a severe complication of active infective endocarditis, commonly caused by *S. aureus*. It can proceed rapidly to valve destruction, myocardial abscess formation, and heart failure. The *Staphylococcus* can affect a completely normal native valve.

The ability of TTE to detect endocarditis is limited. TEE has become an increasingly reliable tool in detecting and evaluating cardiac lesions. In a study, abscess formation, leaflet perforation, noncalcified leaflet thickening, flail chordal structures, and vegetations were found far more often with TEE than with TTE (96% versus 68% for lesions on the aortic valve, and 100% versus 89% for lesions on the mitral valve) [1].

Surgery can be successfully performed during active endocarditis [2]. Patients with active native-valve or prosthetic-valve endocarditis operated on during the course of antibiotic therapy had a relatively low operative mortality. The timing of surgical intervention is very important. Delaying surgery when there is increasing ventricular decompensation may lead to an increase in the rate of mortality. Intracardiac abscesses are rarely cured by antibiotic therapy [3].

An abscess can have several untoward consequences including (1) rupture into the pericardial space; (2) form an intracardiac fistula; (3) worsening AR; and (4) risk of an embolic complication.

References

1. Li JS, Sexton DJ, Mick N, *et al.* Proposed modifications to the Duke criteria for the diagnosis of infective endocarditis. *Clin Infect Dis* 2000;30:633–8.
2. Arnett EN, Roberts WC. Valve ring abscess in active infective endocarditis: frequency, location, and clues to clinical diagnosis from the study of 95 necropsy patients. *Circulation* 1976;54:140–45.
3. Bayer AS, Bolger AF, Taubert KA, *et al.* Diagnosis and management of infective endocarditis and its complications. *Circulation* 1998;98:2936–48.

70 Native Aortic Valve Organized Thrombosis

Jing Ping Sun[1], Xing Sheng Yang[1] & James D. Thomas[2]

[1] Emory University School of Medicine; Emory University Hospital Midtown, Atlanta, GA, USA
[2] The Cleveland Clinic Foundation, Cleveland, OH, USA

History

A 40-year-old woman was admitted with fever and a history of claudication.

Physical Examination

Blood pressure was 132/65 mmHg; pulse was 92/minute. A grade 3/6 systolic ejection and diastole murmur was audible over the aortic ostium.

Laboratory

Echocardiography: M-mode of aortic root from parasternal long-axis view illustrates the thrombi blocking the orifice of aortic leaflets opening and preventing the leaflets from closing, which lead to aortic stenosis and regurgitation. Transthoracic echocardiography (TEE): longitudinal view shows thrombus on the aortic valves. Short-axis view indicates two thrombi on the aortic valvular leaflets (Figure 70.1, Videoclip 70.1). The color Doppler of TEE longitudinal view shows thrombus on the aortic valves causing high-velocity flow through the valve during systole and diastole, which indicates the aortic valvular stenosis and regurgitation (Videoclip 70.2).

Treatment

Aortic valve replacement was performed. Patient recovered well. The pathological diagnosis was aortic valve leaflets with organized thrombus.

Practical Handbook of Echocardiography 1st edition. Edited by Jing Ping Sun, Joel Felner and John Merlino. © 2010 Blackwell Publishing Ltd.

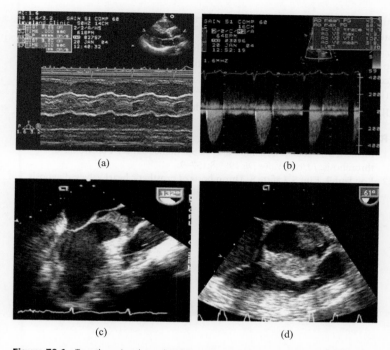

(a)

(b)

(c)

(d)

Figure 70.1. Transthoracic echocardiography: M-mode of aortic root illustrates the thrombi blocking the orifice of aortic leaflets opening and preventing the leaflets from closing (a), which lead to aortic stenosis (b) and regurgitation. Transthoracic echocardiography: longitudinal view shows thrombus on the aortic valves (c), short-axis view indicates two thrombi on the aortic valvular leaflets (d).

Discussion

Native aortic valve thrombus formation is extremely rare. This event occasionally develops after cardiac catheterization, heart valve disease, infective endocarditis or as a hypercoagulative state as in antiphospholipid antibody syndrome. Our case had history of fever and claudication. The thrombi on aortic valve may be a result of infective endocarditis, causing the embolism in the left lower extremity.

This thrombosis may be a result of trauma to the valve endothelium by catheter. Valve dystrophy such as aortic stenosis may induce endothelial lesions, which associated with an abnormal blood flow, may trigger the mechanism of thrombosis [1].

In echocardiogram, aortic thrombosis appeared as masses of echoes attached to the ventricular surface of the leaflets. These echo-producing masses may be smaller or larger, mobile, or fixed and have been described as fuzzy or shaggy in appearance. When the mass is large and mobile, such as our case, the mass may prolapse into left ventricular outflow tract during diastole and may swing forward with the stream of the blood into the aorta during systolic ejection, clinically producing aortic regurgitation and/or stenosis.

Although surgical treatment is usually preferred in cases of obstructive prosthetic valve thrombosis (PVT), optimal treatment remains controversial. The different therapeutic modalities available for PVT (heparin treatment, fibrinolysis, surgery) will be largely influenced by the presence of valvular obstruction, valve location, and clinical status [2].

References

1. Massetti M, Babatasi G, Saloux E, *et al.* Spontaneous native aortic valve thrombosis. *J Heart Valve Dis* 1999;8:157–9.
2. Roudaut R, Kim S, Lafitte S. Thrombosis of prosthetic heart valves: diagnosis and therapeutic considerations. *Heart* 2007;93:137–42.

71 Aortic Valvular Flail Causing Severe Regurgitation

Jing Ping Sun[1], Xing Sheng Yang[1] & Joel M. Felner[2]

[1]Emory University School of Medicine; Emory University Hospital Midtown, Atlanta, GA, USA
[2]Grady Memorial Hospital; Emory University School of Medicine, Atlanta, GA, USA

History

A 50-year-old female presented with fever and severe anterior chest pain. The patient was regularly scheduled for hemodialysis.

Physical Examination

Patient is acutely ill appearing with blood pressure of 164/64 mmHg and heart rate of 96 beats/minute. Grade 3/6 early diastolic decrescendo murmur was heard at the left lower sternal border.

Echocardiogram

Transesophageal echocardiography (TEE) revealed: noncoronary cusp prolapsing into left ventricular outflow tract (LVOT) during diastole and color-flow imaging showed eccentric severe aortic regurgitation (AR) (Figure 71.1 and Videoclip 71.1). M-mode echocardiography in LVOT

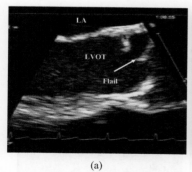
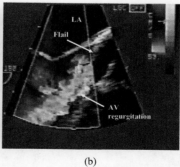

(a)   (b)

Figure 71.1. Transesophageal echocardiography long-axis view showed the flail of noncoronary cusp of aortic valve (a). Color-flow imaging showed eccentric severe aortic regurgitation (b). AV, aortic valve; LA, left atrium; LVOT, left ventricular outflow tract.

Practical Handbook of Echocardiography 1st edition. Edited by Jing Ping Sun, Joel Felner and John Merlino. © 2010 Blackwell Publishing Ltd.

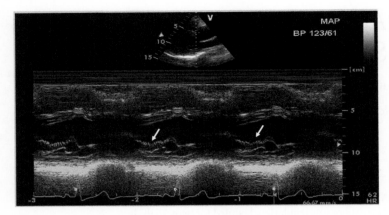

Figure 71.2. M-mode recording of the mitral valve illustrating the high-frequency fluttering (arrows) of the anterior leaflet characteristic of aortic regurgitation due to aortic valvular flail. BP, blood pressure.

demonstrated a high frequency fluttering characteristic (Figure 71.2) of the mitral anterior leaflet caused by AR due to aortic valvular flail. Severe AR was also demonstrated by the flow reversal of color Doppler in the aortic arch (Figure 71.3a), pulse Doppler recording showing the forward and reversal flow in the abdominal aorta (Figure 71.3b), and color M-mode (Figure 71.4).

Hospital Course

Treatment was initiated with high-dose penicillin and gentamicin. Multiple blood cultures were subsequently positive for Streptococcus and

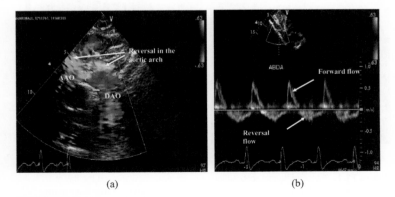

Figure 71.3. Suprasternal notch long-axis view illustrates the reversal flow in the aortic arch (a); pulse Doppler recording shows the forward and reversal flow in the abdominal aorta, which indicates severe aortic regurgitation due to aortic valvular flail (b). AAO, ascending aorta; ABDA, abdomen aorta; DAO, descending aorta.

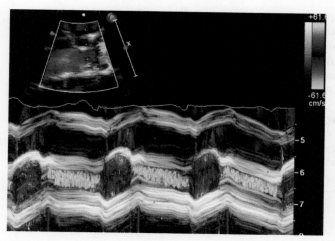

Figure 71.4. M-mode recording of parasternal long-axis view with color Doppler demonstrates the wide opening of aortic closing line and aortic regurgitant flow persistent in the entire diastolic period, which indicates severe aortic regurgitation.

antibiotic therapy was changed to high-dose ampicillin and gentamicin. The patient was thought to have severe acute AR secondary to destruction of aortic noncoronary cusp caused by the endocarditis. He underwent aortic valve replacement. At the time of surgery noncoronary cusp of the aortic valve leaflets was found to have been destroyed by the infection. The postoperative echocardiogram demonstrated disappearance of the abnormal echo patterns in the aortic root and LVOT.

Discussion

Acute AR frequently constitutes a surgical emergency. The recognition of the underlying mechanism and its proper management is crucial in ensuring good outcome. TEE is sensitive for the diagnosis of aortic valve vegetation flail and aortic dissection, the most common causes of acute AR.

Flail aortic valve can be caused by infective endocarditis, aortic dissection, and traumatic rupture of aortic cusps, but rarely by laceration of the ascending aorta [1,2]. Our case was regularly scheduled for hemodialysis and multiple blood cultures were subsequently positive for Streptococcus. The flail aortic valve may be caused by infective endocarditis and was confirmed by surgery.

The echocardiographic manifestations of flail aortic valve leaflet are diastolic fluttering of the aortic cusp echoes and abnormal systolic aortic leaflet movement in LVOT. Both of these echocardiographic characteristics were well seen in our patient. M-mode recording shows characteristic high-frequency fluttering of mitral anterior leaflet. Suprasternal notch long-axis view illustrates the reversal flow in the aortic arch and pulse

Doppler recording shows the forward and reversal flow in the abdominal aorta indicating severe AR.

TEE allows excellent visualization of the aortic valve and ascending aorta. Thus, it is considered to be especially useful in delineating the pathoanatomy of AR. TEE should be considered in patients with chest pain and acute AR.

References

1. Murray CA, Edwards JE. Spontaneous laceration of ascending aorta. *Circulation* 1973;47:848–58.
2. O'Brien KP, Hitchcock GC, Barratt-Boyes BG, *et al*. Spontaneous aortic cusp rupture associated with valvular myxomatous transformation. *Circulation* 1968;37:273–8.

72 Perforation of Aortic Valve due to Bacterial Endocarditis

Xing Sheng Yang[1], Jing Ping Sun[1] & James D. Thomas[2]
[1] Emory University School of Medicine; Emory University Hospital Midtown, Atlanta, GA, USA
[2] The Cleveland Clinic Foundation, Cleveland, OH, USA

History

A 50-year-old female was admitted with a 2-month history of progressive shortness of breath.

Physical Examination

Jugular venous pressure was elevated with a prominent V wave. Auscultation showed gallop, a to-and-fro murmur at left lower sternal border with distinct second sound, a separate ejection systolic murmur at the aortic area, and moist rales in the bilateral lung fields.

Laboratory

X-ray showed mild cardiomegaly with a cardiothoracic ratio of 54% and bilateral pulmonary edema.

Transesophageal echocardiography (TEE): long-axis view of aortic root indicating the aortic valve (right coronary cusp, RCC) prolapse, long-axis view with color Doppler showing aortic valve with severe regurgitation due to prolapse and large perforation in the body of the RCC (Figure 72.1, Videoclip 72.1).

Blood culture grew methicillin-resistant *Staphylococcus aureus*. All these findings supported a diagnosis of infective endocarditis, resulting in aortic valve perforation and regurgitation, accompanied by heart failure.

Discussion

A sinus of Valsalva fistula with left to right shunting from the aorta to right atrium or right ventricle is an unusual complication of infective endocarditis [1].

Aortic valve perforation may occur as the result of various factors which include infective endocarditis, rheumatic change, collagen disease, and

---

Practical Handbook of Echocardiography 1st edition. Edited by Jing Ping Sun, Joel Felner and John Merlino. © 2010 Blackwell Publishing Ltd.

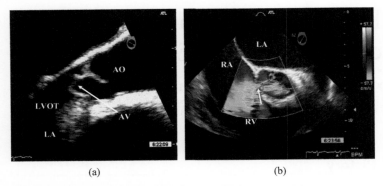

(a)   (b)

Figure 72.1. Transesophageal echocardiography revealed mild thickening of aortic valve with right coronary cusp (RCC) prolapse (a), and trileaflet aortic valve with severe regurgitation due to prolapse and large perforation (arrow) in the body of the RCC (b). AO, aorta; AV, aortic valve; LA, left atrium; LVOT, left ventricular outflow tract; RA, right atrium; RV, right ventricle.

iatrogenic injury such as perforation of the right aortic valve cusp—a complication of ventricular septal defect closure with a modified Rashkind Umbrella [2].

In most cases, the clinical features seemed to be reasonably typical and, when present, have generally been followed by progressive, often intractable heart failure [3].

In this patient, the diagnosis of infective endocarditis was confirmed, complicated with RCC perforation with prolapse resulting in severe aortic regurgitation and heart failure.

Transthoracic echocardiography with color Doppler helps in early and accurate diagnosis ; thus, timely surgical intervention could be undertaken to save patient's life. TEE may be required in a patient with poor echogenicity to depict cardiac structures optimally.

References

1. Seamus C, Sullivan ID. Ruptured sinus of Valsalva with aorta-to-right atrial fistula. *Circulation* 2002; 98:2503–4.
2. Vogel M, Rigby ML, Shore D. Perforation of the right aortic valve cusp: complication of ventricular septal defect closure with a modified Rashkind umbrella. *Pediatr Cardiol* 1996;17:416–18.
3. Tompsett R, Lubash GD. Aortic valve perforation in bacterial endocarditis. *Circulation* 1961;23:662–4.

73 *Bartonella henselae* Endocarditis

John D. Merlino & Jing Ping Sun

Emory University School of Medicine; Emory University Hospital Midtown, Atlanta, GA, USA

History

A 40-year-old male with a past history of fever, bicuspid aortic valve, and myocardial infarction with stent placement.

Echocardiography

Transesophageal echocardiography revealed a 3-cm vegetation on a tricuspid aortic valve. The left ventricle was dilated with mild hypocontractity. Moderate to severe aortic regurgitation was noted (Figure 73.1 and Videoclip 73.1).

(a) (b) (c) (d)

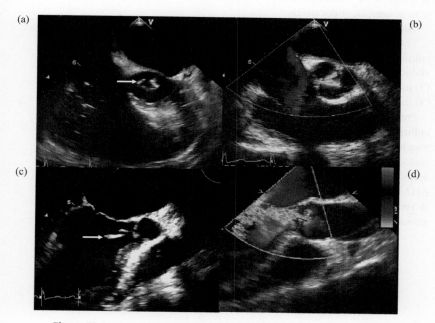

Figure 73.1. Transesophageal echocardiography shows a vegetation (arrow) on the aortic valve (a and c), and aortic regurgitation (b and d).

Practical Handbook of Echocardiography 1st edition. Edited by Jing Ping Sun, Joel Felner and John Merlino. © 2010 Blackwell Publishing Ltd.

Blood cultures were performed but were negative. White blood cell count of 13 K with 70% segs.

Laboratory workup revealed elevation in Bartonella IgG titers of > 1600. PCR of the valve tissue confirming the diagnosis of *Bartonella henselae* endocarditis.

The patient was referred for aortic valve replacement and received a bileaflet mechanical valve without complication. His fever, myalgias, and arthralgias were resolved.

Discussion

The incidence of culture negative endocarditis varies greatly in different countries with reported incidences as low as 6% and as high as 56%. The two most common organisms are *Coxiella burnetti* and various Bartonella species.

Bartonella was first recognized as a cause of endocarditis in 1993. Six species have been identified as causing endocarditis, but over 95% of cases have involved either *Bartonella quintana* or *B. henselae*. Bartonella endocarditis occurs more frequently in men. There appears to be an association with alcoholism, homelessness, and body lice infestation with *B. quintana* infection, and with cat contact and known valvular disease with *B. henselae* endocarditis.

There appears to be a predilection for the aortic valve.

The diagnosis of Bartonella endocarditis is problematic as blood cultures only become positive 25% of the time. Culture negative infective endocarditis occurs for three reasons: (1) prior antibiotic administration; (2) infection with fastidious bacteria or nonbacterial infectious agents; and (3) inadequate technique in the microbiology laboratory.

Preoperative diagnosis requires either the presence of positive blood cultures or elevation in serologic titers. Vegetations are seen on echo roughly 90% of the time. The clinical manifestations of Bartonella endocarditis are little different from other infectious causes. The ideal antibiotic regimen for Bartonella endocarditis is unknown. The current AHA guidelines recommend ceftriaxone and gentamicin with or without doxycycline for suspected Bartonella endocarditis, and doxycycline and gentamicin for confirmed Bartonella endocarditis.

74 A Hydatid Cyst in Left Ventricular Lateral Wall

Yuming Mu[1], Patrick E. BeDell[1] & Jing Ping Sun[2]
[1]XinJiang Medical School, Urumqi, China
[2]Emory University School of Medicine; Emory University Hospital Midtown, Atlanta, GA, USA

History

A 50-year-old male with a one-day history of continuous chest pain along with a history of weakness, fatigue, and shortness of breath.

Physical Examination

Blood pressure was 120/80 mmHg, heart rate was regular at 86 bpm, respiratory rate was 20, and temperature was 36.8°C.

Laboratory

Magnetic resonance imaging demonstrated an infiltrated cystic mass in the lateral region of left ventricle (LV), which was confirmed by subsequent computed tomography.

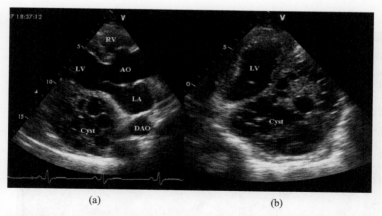

(a)   (b)

Figure 74.1. PLA, Parasternal long axis; shows cyst in the left ventricular posterior wall (a) and posterolateral wall in short-axis view (b). AO, aorta; DAO, descending aorta; LA, left atrium; LV, left ventricle; RV, right ventricle.

Practical Handbook of Echocardiography 1st edition. Edited by Jing Ping Sun, Joel Felner and John Merlino. © 2010 Blackwell Publishing Ltd.

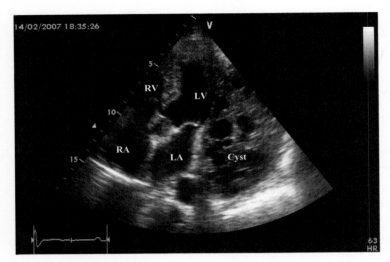

Figure 74.2. Apical 5-chamber shows cyst in left ventricular wall. LA, left atrium; LV, left ventricle; RA, right atrium; RV, right ventricle.

Echocardiography: Multilocular hydatid cyst in LV lateral and posterior wall noted in parasternal long- and short-axis views, which was also seen in apical views (Figures 74.1, 74.2 and Videoclip 74.1, 74.2). The diameter of the mass measured 11 cm. The velocity of lower left pulmonary vein was high (1 m/sec, Figure 74.3 and Videoclip 74.3), caused by mass pressure.

The diagnosis was confirmed with immunohistochemistry and enzyme linked immunosorbent assay for echinococcosis.

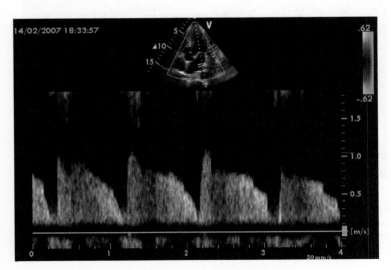

Figure 74.3. The velocity of left low pulmonary vein was 1 m/sec.

Management: Patient underwent surgical resection of the cyst. A multilocular cyst was noted. The cyst consisted of a dense co-liquated material.

Discussion

Heart echinococcosis is uncommon (0.01–2% from all registered echinococcosis cases) [1]. It can occur as part of a widespread systemic infection or as an isolated event. Cardiac hydatid cysts rarely involve the ventricular wall.

Cardiac hydatid cysts can result in serious consequences such as rupture into the circulation with drastic anaphylactic reaction, ischemic syndromes from compression of coronary arteries, conduction abnormalities from bundle compression, heart failure, and systemic or pulmonary embolization [2].

Our case presents with cardiac hydatid disease with a lesion in the LV lateral wall. It was a 10 cm × 9.8 cm^2 tumoral cyst and bulged toward the pericardial cavity. This cyst appeared to be both echolucent and multiseptated. This cyst was clearly demonstrated in multiechocardiographic views.

Two-dimensional echocardiography is a very useful tool for diagnosis. Classic echocardiographic features include the presence of a cystic mass within the myocardium or pericardium that may become calcified with multiple septa and multitextured hypoechoic contents.

Small intramyocardial cysts could be missed by transthoracic echocardiography or transesophageal echocardiography. It is important to perform a complete echocardiogram, including multiple views with careful analysis of all available images.

References

1. Miralles A, Bracamonte L, Pavie A. Cardiac echinococcosis. Surgical treatment and results. *J Thorac Cardiovasc Surg* 1994;107:184–90.
2. Thameur H, Abdelmoula S, Chenic S, *et al.* Cardiopericardial hydatid cysts. *World J Surg* 2001;25:58–67.

75 Acute Endocarditis with Diastolic Mitral Regurgitation

Ambareesh Bajpai & Jing Ping Sun
Emory University School of Medicine; Emory University Hospital Midtown, Atlanta, GA, USA

History

A 30-year-old female complains of fever, chills, and shortness of breath.

Physical Examination

The temperature was 39.2°C, heart rate was 45, blood pressure was 90/30 mmHg, respiratory rate was 40/minute, and O_2 saturation was 84% on 100% FiO_2 by face mask.

Heart revealed holodiastolic murmur.

Laboratory

Electrocardiogram demonstrated complete heart block. Blood culture was positive.

Transthoracic echocardiography: There is aortic and mitral valvular regurgitation during diastole (Figure 75.1a). The Doppler trace shows aortic regurgitation (AR) along with systolic and diastolic mitral regurgitation (MR) (Figure 75.1b).

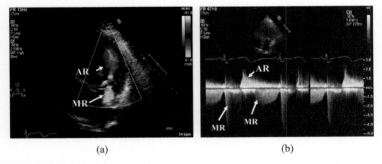

(a)   (b)

Figure 75.1. There is aortic and mitral valvular regurgitation during diastole (a). Doppler trace showed aortic regurgitation, systolic and diastolic mitral regurgitation (b). AR, aortic regurgitation; MR, mitral regurgitation.

Practical Handbook of Echocardiography 1st edition. Edited by Jing Ping Sun, Joel Felner and John Merlino. © 2010 Blackwell Publishing Ltd.

Transesophageal echocardiography images show aortic vegetation, paravalvular abscess, and prolapse; AR, systolic and diastolic MR (Videoclip 75.1).

Discussion

The diagnosis of acute infectious endocarditis (IE) was confirmed in this case. There are two points worthy of discussion on this case—perivalvular abscess formation with heart block and diastolic MR.

Perivalvular extension of endocarditis occurs when the infection breaks through the annulus into the surrounding contiguous tissue. It is relatively common, occurring in 10–40% of cases of native valve IE. Aortic valve endocarditis is more likely to be complicated by periannular extension of infection than mitral or tricuspid valve. In native aortic valve IE, periannular extension of infection is most likely to occur in the weakest portion of the annulus near the membranous septum and aortic valve (AV) node [1]. This anatomic vulnerability explains that this complication is most frequent in patients with aortic valve IE and it is commonly associated with complete heart block.

Diastolic MR occurs as a result of a gradient between the ventricle and atrium in diastole across an incompletely closed mitral valve. It is widely accepted that effective mitral valve closure requires both coordinated and effective atrial and ventricular contraction. Diastolic MR occurs primarily in two settings: (1) AV block of varying degrees; and (2) significantly elevated LV end-diastolic pressures, most often seen in acute severe AR or restrictive ventricular hemodynamics.

In the setting of AV dissociation, the absence of ventricular systole after atrial contraction forces the mitral valve to remain open while atrial relaxation causes a gradient to develop between the ventricle and atrium [2]. In the case of severe acute regurgitation, the mechanism is different and involves the rapid rise of ventricular pressure in diastole due to the AR. This leads to counterintuitive concept of inappropriately early (i.e., presystolic) but functionally incompetent mitral valve closure [3].

In this patient, the combination of AV block and elevated LV end diastolic pressure due to acute severe aortic regurgitation leading to the diastolic MR.

References

1. Baddour LM, Wilson WR, Bayer FV, *et al.* Infective endocarditis: diagnosis, anti-microbial therapy and management of complications. *Circulation* 2005;111:3167–84.
2. Agmon Y, Freeman WK, Oh JK, Seward JB. Diastolic mitral regurgitation. *Circulation* 1999;99:e13.
3. Eusebio J, Louie EK, Edwards LC 3rd, Loeb HS, Scanlon PJ. Alterations in transmitral flow dynamics in patients with early mitral valve closure and aortic regurgitation. *Am Heart J* 1994;128(5):941–7.

76 Infective Endocarditis with Initial Cerebral Abscess and Hemorrhage

Shan Wang, Li-xue Yin, Yan Deng, Ming-liang Zuo, Yang Yu, Zheng-Yang Wang & Shuang Li

Southwest Jiaotong University; Sichuan Academy of Medical Sciences, Sichuan Provincial People's Hospital, Chengdu, Sichuan, China

History

A 16-year-old male was hospitalized because of loss of consciousness with right limb asthenia for 12 hours.

Physical Examination

Regular cardiac rhythm. Grade 3/6 systolic and diastolic murmurs were detected in aortic valve areas. Heart border was enlarged. Muscle strength of the right limb was grade 0.

Laboratory

Electrocardiogram showed sinus tachycardia and T-waves slightly lower in leads V5 and V6. Blood cultures were negative.

Computed tomography (CT) showed irregular shape of hematoma (4.5 $\times$ 4 $\times$ 4.5 cm^3) in the left parietal lobe. The primary diagnosis was cerebral hemorrhage in left parietal lobe.

Transthoracic echocardiography (TTE) revealed an increased end-diastolic diameter of left ventricle (LV) and thickened aortic valve. Echogenic masses were found at LV side of aortic cusps and anterior mitral leaflet. Cord-like echo was found attached at the left side of upper interventricular septum and it swung in LV chamber (Figure 76.1). Vegetations were detected at the endocardium of interventricular septum and aortic valve. An oval hypoechoic area (0.2 cm $\times$ 0.3 cm) was found within the LV basal segment of lateral wall (Figure 76.2). Moderate aortic regurgitation and mitral regurgitation were detected by color Doppler (Figure 76.3).

Practical Handbook of Echocardiography 1st edition. Edited by Jing Ping Sun, Joel Felner and John Merlino. © 2010 Blackwell Publishing Ltd.

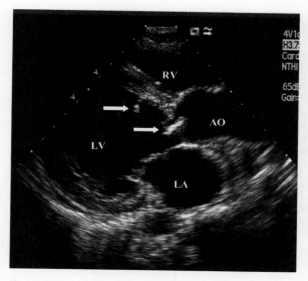

Figure 76.1. Vegetations were detected at the endocardium of interventricular septum and aortic valve (arrows). AO, aorta; LA, left atrium; LV, left ventricle; RV, right ventricle.

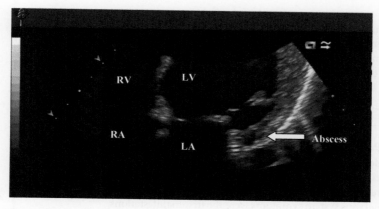

Figure 76.2. Abscess (arrow) at the basal lateral wall of left ventricle. LA, left atrium; LV, left ventricle; RA, right atrium; RV, right ventricle.

Management

The patient received comprehensive treatment but expired because of respiratory and circulatory failure 10 days after admission.

Autopsy Findings

The findings of autopsy: (1) acute infective endocarditis with yellow dirt vegetations, which were attached to aortic, mitral, and tricuspid valve

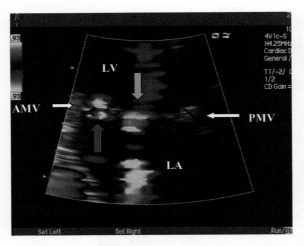

Figure 76.3. Regurgitation jets were detected at the body of anterior leaflet of mitral valve in systole (blue arrow) and also the mitral commissures (green arrow). AMV, anterior mitral leaflet; LA, left atrium; LV, left ventricle; PMV, posterior mitral leaflet.

margins; (2) a perforation at the anterior mitral leaflet; (3) cardiac enlargement; (4) bilateral pulmonary edema; (5) acute purulent meningitis accompanied with abscess formation in brain parenchyma; and (6) multiple organ emboli and abscesses.

Discussion

Patient had fever for several days, and hemorrhage in left parietal lobe was detected by CT, which might be caused by infective endocarditis. Bacterial embolus from exfoliated vegetation reached brain along with blood flow, resulting in cerebral infarction and secondary cerebral hemorrhage. The nervous system symptoms were the first manifestations.

Positive blood culture is important direct evidence in the diagnosis of IE. In a subset of patients (10–25%) with IE, persistently negative blood cultures are noted in spite of active infection [1]. The blood cultures were negative in this patient, but multiple vegetations in the heart, mitral anterior leaflet perforation, and abscesses in the ventricular wall were strongly indicated the diagnosis of infectious endocarditis (IE). TEE is significantly more sensitive and accurate than TTE for small vegetations [2]. There were vegetations in tricuspid valve found by autopsy but not detected by transthoracic echocardiography in this case.

Most available data suggest that patients with clinical endocarditis and echocardiographically detectable vegetations are at increased risk of complications such as systemic emboli, congestive heart failure, and requirement for surgical intervention.

References

1. Gregoraots G, Karliner JS. Infective endocarditis: diagnosis and management. *Med Clin North Am* 1979;63:173.
2. Vieira ML, Grinberg M, Pomerantzeff PM, *et al.* Repeated echocardiographic examinations of patients with suspected infective endocarditis. *Heart* 2004;90:1020.

77 Aortic Root Abscess with Rupture

Xing Sheng Yang[1], Jing Ping Sun[1] & James D. Thomas[2]

[1] Emory University School of Medicine; Emory University Hospital Midtown, Atlanta, GA, USA
[2] The Cleveland Clinic Foundation, Cleveland, OH, USA

History

A 70-year-old man admitted with severe aortic regurgitation and suspected infective endocarditis. He had a history of aortic valve replacement with prosthesis. He had a 2-month history of shortness of breath on exertion. Four sets of blood cultures produced a growth of anaerobic organisms.

Physical Examination

The temperature was 38.0°C, blood pressure was 132/76 mmHg, pulse rate was 98 bpm, and the respiratory rate was 26/minute. Cardiac examination was remarkable for systolic murmur.

Laboratory

Transesophageal echocardiography (TEE) demonstrated a 20×10 mm^2 ruptured aortic-root abscess with a shunt from aortic root to left atrium (Figures 77.1 and 77.2, Videoclip 77.1).

Discussion

Perivalvular abscess is a more common complication of prosthetic than native valve endocarditis. It is not necessarily associated with more virulent microorganisms. If the clinical response to optimum antimicrobial therapy is poor or other signs of uncontrolled sepsis are observed, the diagnosis of abscess formation should be suspected [1]. In a report, aortic-root abscess occurred in 52% of prosthetic valve endocarditis compared with 15% of cases of native valve endocarditis [2]. In an autopsy series of 95 patients with endocarditis, 27 had valve ring abscesses; five clinical clues suggested its presence. The clues were as follows: (a) endocarditis involving the aortic valve; (b) the presence of valvular regurgitation of recent onset;

Practical Handbook of Echocardiography 1st edition. Edited by Jing Ping Sun,
Joel Felner and John Merlino. © 2010 Blackwell Publishing Ltd.

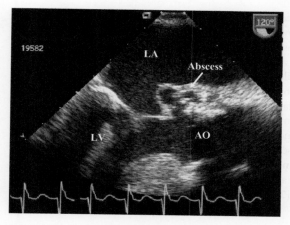

Figure 77.1. Transesophageal echocardiography shows the aortic-root abscess measured at 1 × 2 cm². AO, aorta; LA, left atrium; LV, left ventricle.

(c) evidence of pericarditis; (d) evidence of high-degree atrioventricular block; and (e) a short duration of symptoms caused by endocarditis [3].

In infective endocarditis, spread of infection to surrounding structures is more common with aortic valves. This may result in aortic-root abscess, annular erosion of the aortic root, mycotic aneurysm, or involvement of the aorticomitral apparatus [4].

Echocardiography is helpful in identifying aortic-root abscesses but few patients (<5%) have the obvious finding of an echo-free abscess cavity and thus the diagnosis rests on associated findings such as the wall of the aorta being more than 10 mm thick, prosthetic valve rocking, sinus of Valsalva aneurysm, or perivalvular density in the septum of 14 mm or more. When these factors are considered, the positive and negative predictive values are 86 and 87% respectively [5]. TEE is particularly helpful in diagnosing this

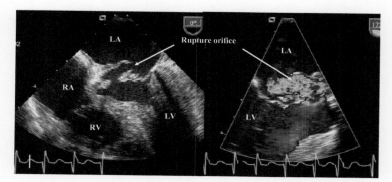

Figure 77.2. Transthoracic echocardiography images show ruptured aortic-root abscess and shunt from aortic root to left atrium. LA, left atrium; LV, left ventricle; RA, right atrium; RV, right ventricle.

complication of infective endocarditis and magnetic resonance imaging may also clearly show an aortic-root abscess [3].

An aortic-root abscess itself does not absolutely indicate the necessity for cardiac surgery [2], and these abscesses have occasionally healed with medical treatment alone [3]. One patient with endocarditis of a prosthetic aortic valve caused by three anaerobic organisms (based on positive blood cultures) was associated with an aortic-root abscess; he was placed on a 6-week regimen of metronidazole. His fever quickly resolved, and he remained healthy and asymptomatic at 8 months. Serial echocardiography showed that the abscess decreased in size from 15 to 12 mm [3]. When surgery was performed, the mortality rate was significantly higher in those with an aortic-root abscess (13.6% compared with 2.2% for those without this complication) [2].

References

1. Lee PYC, Martin MJ, Treasure T. Propionibacterium acnes causing perivalve abscess. *Heart* 1993;69:470–72.
2. John RM, Pugsley W, Treasure T, *et al.* Aortic root complications of infective endocarditis influence on surgical outcome. *Eur Heart J* 1991;12:241–8.
3. Jeang MK, Fuentes F, Gately A, *et al.* Aortic root abscess: initial experience using magnetic resonance imaging. *Chest* 1986;89:613–15.
4. Horner SM, Sturridge MF, Swanton RH. Propionibacterium acnes causing an aortic root abscess. *Br Heart J* 1992;68:218–20.
5. Ellis SG, Goldstein J, Popp RL. Detection of endocarditis associated perivalvular abscess by two dimensional echocardiography. *J Am Coll Cardiol* 1985;5:647–53.

78 *Aspergillus* Pacemaker Endocarditis

Xing Sheng Yang[1], Jing Ping Sun[1] & James D. Thomas[2]

[1] Emory University School of Medicine; Emory University Hospital Midtown, Atlanta, GA, USA
[2] The Cleveland Clinic Foundation, Cleveland, OH, USA

History

An 18-year-old male presented with cyanotic episodes of chills and shaking. He had a history of viral myocarditis leading to pacemaker implant 3 years ago.

Physical Examination

The temperature was 37.8°C; the pulse rate was 92/minute. Cardiac examination and chest X-ray film were unremarkable. He had a right ankle ring-like skin lesion that thought to be aspergillus fungal infection. There were no inflammatory signs at the pacemaker pocket.

Laboratory

Transthoracic echocardiography and transesophageal echocardiography showed a large vegetation attached to his pacemaker wires (Figure 78.1, Videoclip 78.1). The interventricular septal was flat (D pattern) during

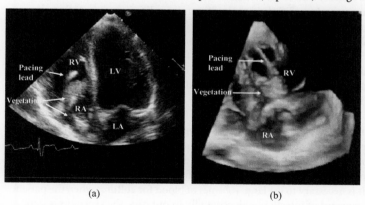

(a)   (b)

Figure 78.1. Apical 4-chamber view shows the pacing lead and a large vegetation by two-dimensional (a) and three-dimensional echocardiography (b). LA, left atrium; LV, left ventricle; RA, right atrium; RV, right ventricle.

Practical Handbook of Echocardiography 1st edition. Edited by Jing Ping Sun, Joel Felner and John Merlino. © 2010 Blackwell Publishing Ltd.

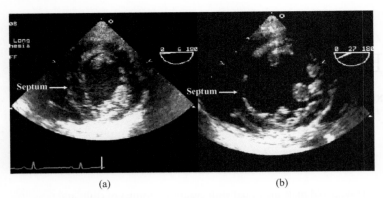

(a)   (b)

Figure 78.2. The interventricular septal was flat (D pattern) during systole and diastole from the parasternal short-axis view (a). Post operation, the shape of ventricular septum recovered to normal pattern (b).

systole and diastole from parasternal short axis view, which returned to normal after operation (Figure 78.2). Pacemaker was removed. Post operation, the tricuspid valve recovered to normal pattern (Videoclip 78.2).

The vegetations were cultured and found with aspergillus growth.

Discussion

The fungal endocarditis is a rare disease, with fungi responsible for less than 10% of the cases with infective endocarditis fungal endocarditis is a rare disease, with fungi responsible for less than 10% of the cases with infective endocarditis [1]. *Aspergillus* endocarditis in man usually occurs on prosthetic cardiac valves and gives rise to large vegetations which embolize easily producing peripheral organ infarction and infection. Pacemaker implantation may be a risk factor for the development of fungal endocarditis [2]. Other risk factors for developing fungal endocarditis include indwelling catheters, prolonged antibiotic therapy, malignancy, and intravenous drug use [3].

Aspergillus endocarditis was studied in rabbits; polyethylene tubing was introduced into the left ventricle through the carotid artery and 24 hours later animals were inoculated with spores of a strain of *Aspergillus fumigatus*. Large occlusive vegetations developed on the aortic valves. Spontaneous mortality reached 67% after 3 days [4].

It is necessary to get large volumes of blood for cultures when the patient is suspected of infection with aspergilli. In our case, the vegetations were cultured and found to grow aspergillus, but blood cultures were negative.

The diagnosis of fungal endocarditis requires a high index of clinical suspicion. Echocardiography usually shows a large vegetation attached to the pacemaker wires or on prosthetic cardiac valves. Aspergilli grew in the blood only when large volumes were cultured.

Over the past decade, the clinical development of several new compounds and strategies targeted against invasive aspergillosis have occurred. Our patient underwent a successful surgery to remove the infected pacemaker wire and was discharged on chronic antifungal therapy.

References

1. Ellis M, Al-Abdely H, Sandridge A, *et al.* Fungal endocarditis. Evidence in the world literature 1965–1995. *Clin Infect Dis* 2001;32:50–62.
2. Leong R, Gannon BR, Childs TJ, *et al. Aspergillus fumigatus* pacemaker lead endocarditis: a case report and review of the literature. *Can J Cardiol* 2006;15:337–40.
3. El-Hamamsy I, Dürrleman N, Stevens LM, *et al.* Aspergillus endocarditis after cardiac surgery. *Ann Thorac Surg* 2005;80:359–64.
4. Carrizosa J, Kohn C, Levison ME. Experimental aspergillus endocarditis in rabbits. *J Lab Clin Med* 1975;86:746–53.

79 Mitral Leaflet Perforation Secondary to Infective Endocarditis

Xing Sheng Yang, Jing Ping Sun & Byron R. Williams, Jr.

Emory University School of Medicine; Emory University Hospital Midtown, Atlanta, GA, USA

History

A 50-year-old female complains of increasing sternal drainage from the most inferior portion of her median sternotomy. She has a history of coronary artery bypass 20 days ago.

Physical Examination

Temperature was 38.5°C, blood pressure was 120/82 mmHg, heart rate was 95/minute, and respiratory rate was 28/minute. Except for the incision that was carried down through subcutaneous tissue, the physical exam was essentially unremarkable.

Laboratory

Laboratory results: hematocrit was 34, hemoglobin 11.4 g, and WBC 8100/mm^3. Transesophageal echocardiography (TEE) and transthoracic echocardiography (TTE) revealed moderately dilated left atrium; aortic valve is sclerotic. A 1.5-cm vegetation on the mitral posterior valve leaflet, consistent with endocarditis and severe mitral regurgitation (MR) (Figure 79.1, Videoclip 79.1). TEE image with color Doppler shows two jets of MR, one through mitral leaflets coaptation, another anterior direction jet from the mitral posterior leaflet perforation (Figure 79.2).

Magnetic resonance image found two jets of regurgitation consistent with TEE image (Figure 79.3, Videoclip 79.2). Culture was obtained from the incision. This grew out 1+ coagulase-negative Staphylococcus (not *Staphylococcus aureus*).

Practical Handbook of Echocardiography 1st edition. Edited by Jing Ping Sun, Joel Felner and John Merlino. © 2010 Blackwell Publishing Ltd.

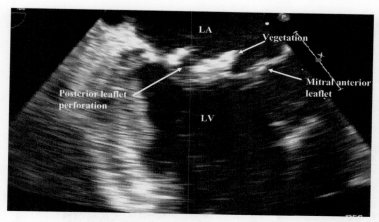

Figure 79.1. Transesophageal image shows the perforation (long arrow) and a vegetation of mitral posterior leaflet. LA, left atrium; LV, left ventricle.

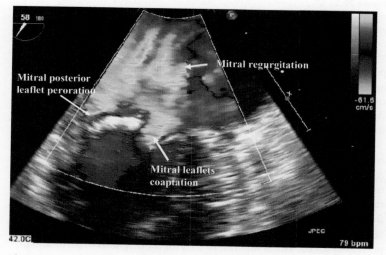

Figure 79.2. Transesophageal echocardiography image with color Doppler (systole) shows two jets of mitral regurgitation, one through mitral leaflets coaptation, another anterior direction jet from the mitral posterior leaflet perforation.

Discussion

Mitral valve perforation is a rare complication of bacterial endocarditis; however, with the use of newer imaging tools such as TEE and real-time 3D echocardiography, the incidence may be higher than previously reported. The perforation rates were 8–20% in autopsy studies. The frequency estimated using TEE imaging is as high as 34–61%, in patients with a history of endocarditis. The mechanisms resulting in mitral leaflet

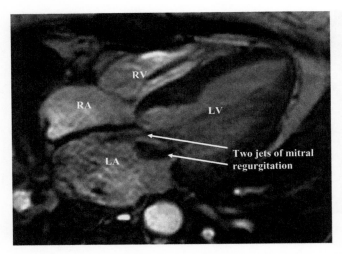

Figure 79.3. Magnetic resonance image illustrates two jets of regurgitation, one through mitral leaflets coaptation, another anterior direction jet from the mitral posterior leaflet perforation. LA, left atrium; LV, left ventricle; RA, right atrium; RV, right ventricle.

perforation include (1) primary leaflet destruction caused by the infectious agent; (2) direct extension from aortic valve endocarditis; (3) continuous impingement of aortic regurgitation jet on the mitral valve leaflet causing disruption; and (4) altered leaflet anatomic structure as a result of prior infective endocarditis [1].

Identification of the cause of MR is important for management and subsequent surgical approach. Two-dimensional echocardiography with color Doppler may raise the suggestion of leaflet perforation when the mosaic-colored flow acceleration appears to traverse the mitral leaflet rather than originating from the leaflet coaptation site. Visualization of the frame with the maximal MR jet, with and without color Doppler, may reveal the discontinuity in the leaflet tissue at the site of the perforation. As previously stated, TEE is superior to TTE for the diagnosis of perforation, with higher sensitivity (95%) and specificity (98%) rates [2,3].

Three-dimensional TEE approach in endocarditis has been reported to have sensitivity and specificity that range between 67–100% and 78–100% for the anterior leaflet and 100% sensitivity and specificity for the posterior leaflet. The diagnostic capability of this technique varies depending on the leaflet segment or scallop involved. In the same study, the correspondence between 3D TEE images and operative findings was excellent [4]. The capability of the surgeon to review the 3D images before operation allows assessment of the feasibility of repair.

References

1. Yanez Wonenburger JC, Garcia-Fernandez MA, San Roman Snachez D, *et al.* Perforation of the mitral valve transesophageal echocardiographic diagnosis in 3 cases. *Rev Esp Cardiol* 1994;47:56–9.

2. Cziner DG, Rosenzweig BP, Katz ES, *et al.* Transesophageal versus transthoracic echocardiography for diagnosing mitral valve perforation. *Am J Cardiol* 1992;69:1495–7.
3. De Castro S, Cartoni D, d'Amati G, *et al.* Diagnostic accuracy of transthoracic and multiplane transesophageal echocardiography for valvular perforation in acute infective endocarditis correlation with anatomic findings. *Clin Infect Dis* 2000;30:825–6.
4. Kanzaki Y, Yoshida K, Hozumi T, *et al.* Evaluation of mitral valve lesions in patients with infective endocarditis by three-dimensional echocardiography. *J Cardiol* 1999;33:7–11.

Part 10
Cardiomyopathy

.

Part 10

Cardiomyopathy

80 Hypertrophic Cardiomyopathy

Jing Ping Sun, Xing Sheng Yang & John D. Merlino

Emory University School of Medicine, Emory University Hospital Midtown, Atlanta, GA, USA

Hypertrophic cardiomyopathy (HCM) is a disease characterized by marked hypertrophy of ventricles, involving in particular the interventricular septum and left ventricular outflow tract (LVOT).

Echocardiography has been used extensively in diagnosis of HCM. The apical 4- and 2-chamber images obtained from transthoracic echocardiography showed the variation of asymmetric left ventricle (LV) hypertrophic cardiomyopathy: ventricular septum, papillary muscle, apical and inferior wall hypertrophy (Figure 80.1).

Figure 80.2 illustrates: The narrow LVOT causing the premature closure (arrow) of aortic leaflets. Systolic anterior motion (SAM) during systole by M-mode recording from aortic root and mitral inflow in a case with interventricular septum hypertrophy. Different shapes of continuous wave Doppler from LVOT are important indicators for diagnosis; normal is symmetric (Figure 80.2c) and asymmetric indicates obstruction of LVOT (Figure 80.2d). Three-dimensional echocardiography demonstrates the narrow LVOT and SAM (Figure 80.3).

SAM consists of varying components, which can be mitral anterior leaflet, bileaflets, or posterior leaflet (Figure 80.4).

The blood flow through the narrow tract, due to venturi effect, sucking mitral leaflets into LVOT and causing the gradient are shown in Figure 80.5.

In the case with HCM, an echocardiographer should measure the distance between SAM contact and basal of septal, maximal septal bulge before and post myectomy or ablation (Figure 80.6).

Videoclip 80.1 demonstrates different types of hypertrophic cardiomyopathy: (a) apical 5-chamber views show the basal septal hypertrophy causing SAM; (b) the obstruction in the mid cavity of LV; (c) color Doppler image shows high-velocity flow through LVOT and posterior direction MR; and (d) apical hypertrophy spade-like pattern.

Treatments for hypertrophic cardiomyopathy, depending on the heart condition and the severity of symptoms, are intended to decrease the stress on the heart and relieve symptoms. Medications help relax the heart and reduce the degree of obstruction so the heart can pump more efficiently. Myectomy is the surgical removal of part of the overgrown septal muscle to decrease LVOT obstruction.

Practical Handbook of Echocardiography 1st edition. Edited by Jing Ping Sun, Joel Felner and John Merlino. © 2010 Blackwell Publishing Ltd.

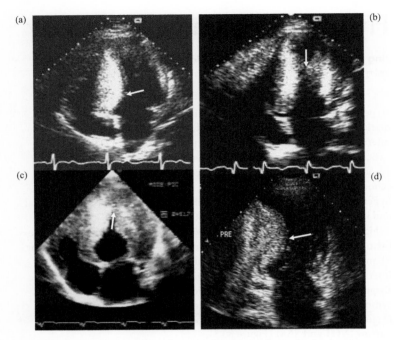

Figure 80.1. Transthoracic echocardiography: Apical 4-chamber and 2-chamber views show the variation of asymmetric left ventricle hypertrophic cardiomyopathy: ventricular septum (arrow, a), papillary muscle (arrow, b), apical (arrow, c) and inferior (arrow, d) wall hypertrophy.

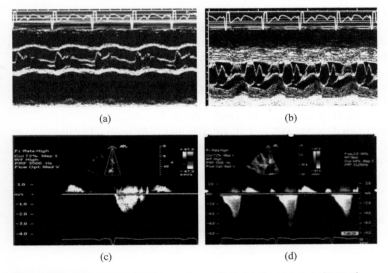

Figure 80.2. M-mode recording from aortic root illustrates: the premature closure of aortic leaflets (a), the mitral anterior leaflet anterior motion during systole (systolic anterior motion) (b). Different shapes of continues wave Doppler from left ventricular outflow tract are important indicators for diagnosis; normal is symmetric (c) and asymmetric indicates the obstruction of left ventricular outflow tract (d).

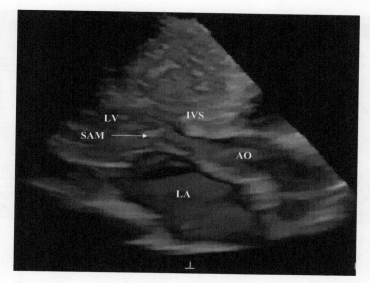

Figure 80.3. Apical 3-chamber of the three-dimensional image illustrates the thickened septum caused left ventricular outflow tract stenosis and systolic anterior mitral leaflet anterior motion (arrow). AO, aorta; IVS, interventricular septum; LA, left atrium; LV, left ventricle; SAM, systolic anterior motion.

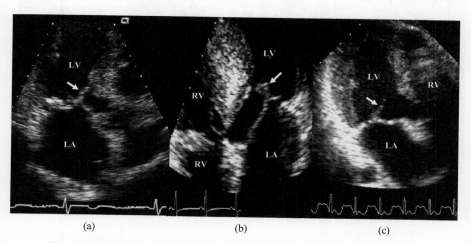

(a)   (b)   (c)

Figure 80.4. The sign of systolic anterior motion of mitral leaflet is vary, which can be mitral anterior leaflet (arrow, a), bileaflets (arrow, b) or posterior leaflet (arrow, c). LA, left atrium; LV, left ventricle; RV, right ventricle.

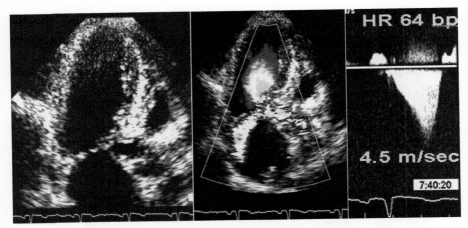

Figure 80.5. These images show the example of venturi effect sucking of mitral leaflets into the narrow left ventricular outflow tract and causing the gradient.

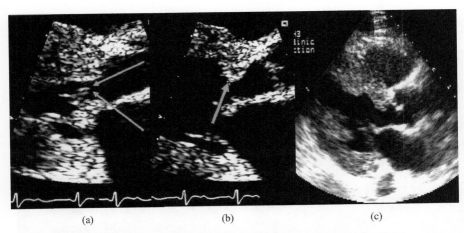

(a)   (b)   (c)

Figure 80.6. Echocardiographer should measure the distance between systolic anterior motion contact and basal of septal (arrow, a), maximal septal bulge (arrow, b) before and post myectomy (c) or ablation.

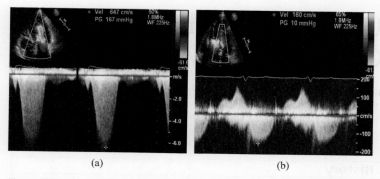

(a)   (b)

Figure 80.7. Continuous wave Doppler recording demonstrates the gradient through obstructed left ventricular outflow tract was 167 mmHg before percutaneous alcohol septal ablation (a) and recovered to 10 mmHg after ablation (b).

Thickened septal ablation is a new technique in which an alcohol solution is injected into an artery supplying the part of the thickened muscle causing the obstruction. The result is a localized "heart attack" of this region of the heart muscle and will decrease the degree of obstruction. Continuous wave Doppler recording demonstrated the gradient through obstructed LVOT was 167 mmHg before percutaneous alcohol septal ablation and recovered to 10 mmHg after ablation in one of our cases (Figure 80.7).

81 Unusual Hypertrophy Cardiomyopathy

Jing Ping Sun[1], Alicia N. Rangosch[1] & Joel M. Felner[2]
[1] Emory University School of Medicine; Emory University Hospital Midtown, Atlanta, GA, USA
[2] Grady Memorial Hospital; Emory University School of Medicine, Atlanta, GA, USA

History

A 25-year-old male complained of chest pain due to his defibrillator firing five times that morning. He had a history of ventricular tachycardia, had an implanted cardioverter defibrillator implanted at 22 years of age, and had a ventricular septal defect repaired in childhood.

Physical Examination

Blood pressure was 121/56 mmHg, heart rate was 76/minute, and respiration rate was 20/minute. Cardiovascular examination: regular rate.

Laboratory

Electrocardiogram: Normal sinus rhythm, incomplete right bundle block, left ventricular hypertrophy (LVH), ST depress in II, III, AVF leads and T wave inverted in I, AVL leads.

Echocardiography: The left ventricle (LV) is normal in systolic function. Apical 4-, 2-chamber, parasternal short-axis, and right ventricle (RV) inflow views show LV lateral (1.6 cm), anterior (2.0 cm), inferior (2.0 cm), and RV free walls (0.9 cm) are significantly thickened. The interventricular septal (0.9 cm) and posterior walls (1.1 cm) were normal (Figures 81.1 and 81.2, Videoclip 80.1).

The left atrium and right atrium are normal in size and structure. Mild tricuspid regurgitation is detected. The tricuspid regurgitant velocity is 2.93 m/sec, and the estimated pulmonary artery systolic pressure is moderately elevated (44.3 mmHg).

Pulse Doppler from mitral valve, pulse tissue Doppler from mitral annulus septal corner and color M-mode recordings show E/E′ = 15.4 and

---

Practical Handbook of Echocardiography 1st edition. Edited by Jing Ping Sun, Joel Felner and John Merlino. © 2010 Blackwell Publishing Ltd.

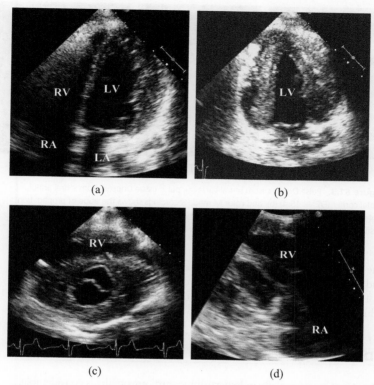

Figure 81.1. Transthoracic echocardiography: apical 4-chamber (a), 2-chamber (b), parasternal short-axis (c) and right ventricle inflow (d) views show left ventricle lateral (1.6 cm), anterior (2.0 cm), inferior (2.0 cm), and right ventricle free walls (0.9 cm) are significantly thickened. LA, left atrium; LV, left ventricle; RA, right atrium; RV, right ventricle.

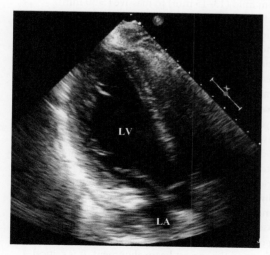

Figure 81.2. Transthoracic echocardiography: apical long-axis view shows the ventricular anterior septal and posterior wall are normal in thickness. LA, left atrium; LV, left ventricle.

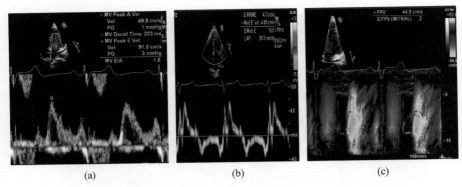

(a)   (b)   (c)

Figure 81.3. Pulse Doppler from mitral valve (a), pulse tissue Doppler from mitral annulus septal corner (E/E′ = 15.4) (b), and color M-mode recordings shows the slope of propagation = 44.5 cm/sec. (c) These results indicate that the 25-year-old young man with diastolic dysfunction.

the slope of color M-mode = 44.5 cm/sec (Figure 81.3). These results indicate a 25-year-old young man with diastolic dysfunction.

His pacing lead was misfiring due to one wire with slight fragmentation, which was repaired.

Discussion

Structural heterogenicity in hypertrophic cardiomyopathy is considerable, with no single pattern of LVH regarded as typical [1]. *LV septal hypertrophy is the most common type of asymmetrical hypertrophy.* Increased LV wall thickness in patients with hypertrophic cardiomyopathy (HCM) range widely from mild (13–15 mm) to massive (>30 mm).

The diagnosis of HCM is established most reliably by echocardiography showing the hypertrophied, but nondilated LV in the absence of hypertension, aortic stenosis, and amyloidosis.

Our patient had an unusual distribution of hypertrophy localized to LV lateral, anterior, and inferior walls, as well as RV free wall. These unusual forms of HCM, in contrast to LVOT contraction type, may be characterized by minor cardiovascular symptoms and a generally benign prognosis. The cardiomyopathic process in HCM is not only confined to areas of wall hypertrophy. Even nonhypertrophied regions may contribute to ischemia or impaired diastolic function. Disorganized cellular architecture and myocardial scarring are arrhythmogenic and predisposing to life-threatening electrical instability [2]. This is likely the source of primary ventricular tachycardia and ventricular fibrillation, which appear to be the predominant mechanisms of sudden cardiac death [3].

Echocardiographic assessment of a patient with HCM requires comprehensive imaging of multiple views. The PLA axis view is of pivotal importance for orientation and the correct beam alignment. It is critical that the beam transects LV perpendicularly, because oblique images will lead to the overestimation of wall thickness and cavity dimensions. Diagnostic features can be missed with an incomplete echocardiographic evaluation.

References

1. Maron BJ. Hypertrophic cardiomyopathy. *Lancet* 1997;350:127–33.
2. St. John Sutton MG, Lie JT, Anderson KR, *et al.* Histopathological specificity of hypertrophic obstructive cardiomyopathy. *Br Heart J* 1980;44:433–44.
3. Maron BJ, Shen W-K, Link MS, *et al.* Efficacy of implantable cardioverter-defibrillators for the prevention of sudden death in patients with hypertrophic cardiomyopathy. *N Engl J Med* 2000;342:365–73.

82 Transcoronary Ablation of Septal Hypertrophy in Hypertrophic Obstructive Cardiomyopathy

Yuhai Ho & Zhi An Li

Beijing Anzhen Hospital, Capital Medical University, Beijing, China

History

A 42-year-old male presented with a 1-year history of exercise-induced chest pain.

Physical examination: Blood pressure was 130/85 mmHg. Apical impulse was located at the left fifth intercostal space, 1 cm lateral to the midclavicular line. A grade 5/6 murmur and a grade 3/6 murmur were heard at the aortic auscultation area and at the mitral auscultation area, respectively.

Laboratory

Chest X-ray showed a cardiothoracic ratio of 60%.

Echocardiogram shows an asymmetric hypertrophy of left ventricular (LV) wall—the thickness of septal basal segment was 21 mm, the middle segment was 17 mm, and the posterior wall was 12 mm. left atrium was dilated. Systolic anterior motion (SAM) sign was positive. Mitral valve was structurally normal with moderate regurgitation. Pulse wave Doppler and continuous wave Doppler (CW) showed that the location of acceleration of left ventricular outflow tract (LVOT) flow was at mitral tip level. LVOT max velocity was 4 m/sec by CW. Pulse Doppler revealed LV diastolic dysfunction at stage II.

Transcoronary ablation of septal hypertrophy (TASH) procedure: Color Doppler coronary flow imaging revealed coronary septal branch in the hypertrophic septum. Based on the order of septal branches, the second branch was confirmed as target vessel (Figure 82.1), which was confirmed by perioperative coronary angiography.

Echocardiography-guided TASH: Before TASH, target vessel was determined and ablated myocardium was quantitated by myocardial

Practical Handbook of Echocardiography 1st edition. Edited by Jing Ping Sun, Joel Felner and John Merlino. © 2010 Blackwell Publishing Ltd.

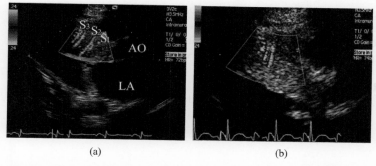

(a)   (b)

Figure 82.1. Doppler coronary flow imaging: The second branch was confirmed as target vessel (a). The second branch disappeared after ablation (b). AO, aorta; LA, left atrium.

contrast. After TASH, the region of perfusion defect was matched with the region of perfusion territory of target vessel (Figure 82.2).

Post-procedure, the pressure gradient in LVOT was reduced more than 50% (from 64 to 20 mmHg).

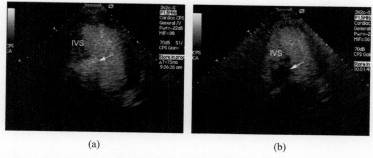

(a)   (b)

Figure 82.2. Contrast agent was injected into left anterior descending coronary artery before (a) and after transcoronary ablation of septal hypertrophy (b). The local infarction region is consistent with the perfusion territory of the second branch. IVS, interventricular septum.

Discussion

Echocardiography plays an important role in the selection of therapeutic strategies, evaluation of effect, and long-term follow-up in patients with hypertrophic obstructive cardiomyopathy. The methods of management for hypertrophic cardiomyopathy (HCM) include medical conservative treatment, surgical treatment for excising hypertrophic myocardium, mitral valve replacement, and implantation of pacemaker. Percutaneous septal myocardial ablation was first introduced by Sigwart in 1995 [1]. There must be a septal branch as target vessel for ablation when performing TASH. Until recently, there was no noninvasive technique to select the target vessel. We used color Doppler coronary flow imaging to select the target coronary septal branch combined with myocardial contrast guiding the TASH procedure in cases with HCM. It is a noninvasive tool used to select a target vessel for ablation and follow-up.

Reference

1. Sigwart U. Non-surgical myocardial reduction for hypertrophic obstructive cardiomyopathy. *Lancet* 1995;346:211–14.

83 Primary Endocardial Fibroelastosis

Jing Ping Sun[1], Xing Sheng Yang[1] & James D. Thomas[2]

[1] Emory University School of Medicine; Emory University Hospital Midtown, Atlanta, GA, USA
[2] The Cleveland Clinic Foundation, Cleveland, OH, USA

History

A 30-year-old male complains of a 6-month history of progressive shortness of breath and edema of lower extremities.

Physical Examination

Blood pressure was 124/76 mmHg and neck revealed vein distention. Cardiac examination documented P2 increase with no significant murmur, rubs, or clicks. Lungs revealed bibasilar rales and abdomen revealed hepatomegaly. There was a grade 4+ edema of the lower extremities.

Laboratory

Electrocardiogram showed a normal sinus rhythm with non-specific ST and T wave changes.

Chest X-ray revealed a mild cardiomegaly with upper zone redistribution.

Catheterization: Coronary arteries were normal.

Echocardiogram showed diffuse hyperplasia of left ventricle (LV) endocardium and systolic dysfunction (Figure 83.1 and Videoclip 83.1), moderate mitral regurgitation.

Patient underwent endocardial resection and mitral replacement, the echocardiographic images shown in Videoclip 83.2.

Discussion

The term endocardial fibroelastosis (EFE) was introduced by Weinberg and Himmelfarb in 1943 [1]. EFE refers to a pronounced, diffuse thickening of the ventricular endocardium and presents as unexplained heart failure. This disorder may be primary and secondary. The primary form is not associated with any congenital cardiac defects and involves the LV almost

Practical Handbook of Echocardiography 1st edition. Edited by Jing Ping Sun, Joel Felner and John Merlino. © 2010 Blackwell Publishing Ltd.

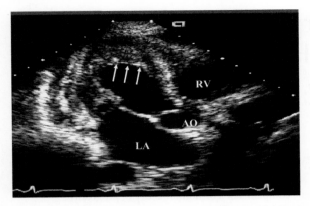

Figure 83.1. Apical long-axis view of a patient with endocardial fibroelastosis illustrates the diffuse hyperplasia of the endocardium and the highly reflective layer in the apical area (arrows). AO, aorta; LA, left atrium; RV, right ventricle.

exclusively [2]; our case is consistent with primary form. Primary endocardial fibroelastosis can be subdivided on the basis of LV size into the dilated and contracted forms [3]. The dilated form, in which the ventricular chamber is enlarged and the wall is thickened, is more common. The aortic and mitral valves also can be involved; the fibrosed and thickening valves may lead to regurgitation.

Secondary EFE is pathologically indistinguishable from the primary form. In general, however, the secondary variety is of a more focal nature, and the endocardial proliferation is less marked. The symptoms of endocardial fibroelastosis are related to the overgrowth of fibrous tissues causing cardiac hypertrophy, especially the LV. Impaired heart and lung function eventually lead to congestive heart failure.

Complications included resistant cardiac failure, recurrent chest infections, and severe failure to thrive. Early diagnosis and prompt persistent administration of digitalis may result in clinical improvement and reversion of cardiac enlargement to normal. The prognosis is relatively poor, although the condition is not universally fatal. It will be worse if onset of heart failure occurs earlier.

References

1. Weinberg T, Himmelfarb AJ. Endocardial fibroelastosis. *Bull Johns Hopkins Hosp* 1943;72:299.
2. Manning JA, Keith JD. Fibroelastosis in children. *Prog Cardiovasc Dis* 1964;7:172.
3. Moller JH, Lucas RV Jr, Adams P Jr, Anderson RC, Jorgens J, Edwards JE. Endocardial fibroelastosis. A clinical and anatomic study of 47 patients with emphasis on its relationship to mitral insufficiency. *Circulation* 1964;30:759–82.

84 Cardiac Amyloidosis

Jing Ping Sun & Dan Sorescu

Emory University School of Medicine; Emory University Hospital Midtown, Atlanta, GA, USA

History

Case 1: A 50-year-old male complains of increased fatigue, lower-extremity edema, and has a history of syncope.

Case 2: A 60-year-old woman presents with congestive heart failure.

Physical Examination

Case 1: Temperature was 37.1°C, blood pressure was 109/76 mmHg, heart rate was 109/minute, and respiratory rate was 20/minute. Jugular vein pressure was at 12 cm. Normal S1, S2 with irregular heartbeat. No audible murmurs. Lower extremities trace edema and warmth.

Case 2: Temperature was 36.8°C, blood pressure was 110/70 mmHg, heart rate was 112/minute, respiratory rate was 24/minute. Jugular vein pressure was at 14 cm. Normal S1, S2 with regular heart rate. There was a 2/6 systolic murmur.

Laboratory

Case 1: There were persistent atrial flutter and paroxysmal ventricular tachycardia documented by Holter monitor. Catheterization revealed normal coronaries free of disease. Cardiac amyloidosis was confirmed by biopsy.

Echocardiography showed that left ventricle (LV) cavity size was normal with moderate hypertrophy. (Figure 84.1). LV ejection fraction (EF) was 50%. Left atrium was mildly dilated. Right ventricle cavity size was normal with mild hypertrophy with borderline systolic function. The mitral valvular leaflets were mildly thickened with trace MR with no evidence of mitral valve stenosis. Spectral Doppler showed pseudonormal pattern of LV diastolic filling (Figure 84.2).

The aortic valve was trileaflet and structurally normal. The tricuspid and pulmonic valves were normal in structure and function. Trace tricuspid regurgitation was detected. The tricuspid regurgitant velocity was 2.52 m/sec; the estimated pulmonary artery systolic pressure was normal at 30.4 mmHg. A small pericardial effusion was present.

Practical Handbook of Echocardiography 1st edition. Edited by Jing Ping Sun, Joel Felner and John Merlino. © 2010 Blackwell Publishing Ltd.

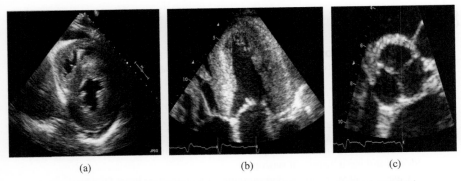

(a)   (b)   (c)

Figure 84.1. Left ventricular and right ventricular wall thickness was moderately increased in case 1 (a). The thickness of left ventricular wall and mitral leaflets was significantly increased (b); the aortic valvular annular and leaflets were thickened (c) in case 2.

Case 2: Echocardiogram showed a severe concentric LV hypertrophy with restrictive diastolic dysfunction (Figure 84.3 b,c and Videoclip 84.1). Assessment of long-axis contraction using 2D strain imaging showed severe impairment in longitudinal strain, even the LV EF was within

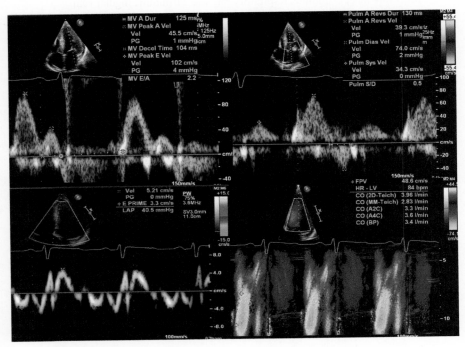

Figure 84.2. Doppler recordings of mitral valvular inflow, pulmonary vein inflow, pulse tissue Doppler, and the color M-mode indicated the pseudo normal pattern of diastolic dysfunction in case 1.

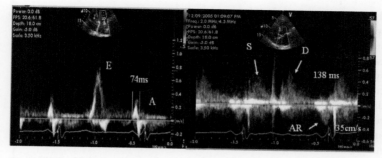

Figure 84.3. Doppler recordings of mitral valvular inflow and pulmonary vein inflow indicated the restrictive pattern of diastolic dysfunction in case 2. AR, atrial reversal.

normal range (Figure 84.4). Cardiac catheterization showed normal coronary arteries. Cardiac biopsy showed amyloid deposits. Despite treatment with melphalan, prednisone, and adequate cardiac therapy, the patient died 8 months after the diagnosis of multiple myeloma due to intractable congestive heart failure.

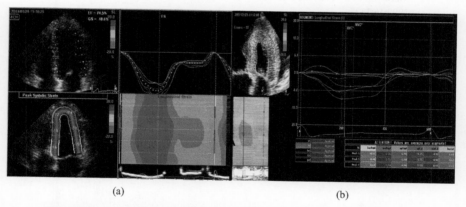

(a)   (b)

Figure 84.4. Longitudinal strain is synchronized and higher in a normal person (a). Longitudinal strain is significantly reduced in case 2 with cardiac amyloidosis (b).

Discussion

Amyloidosis refers to the extracellular tissue deposition of fibrils that are composed of low molecular weight subunits of a variety of serum proteins. Amyloid deposits can occur in a variety of organs. Cardiac involvement is common. Amyloidosis is reported to account for 5–10% of noncoronary cardiomyopathies [1].

The classic echocardiographic feature of cardiac amyloidosis is left and/or right ventricular wall thickening with evidence of diastolic dysfunction and is typically symmetric with a speckled or granular sparkling appearance and normal or small cavity [2]. In more advanced stages of disease, wall thickening progresses, resulting in a restrictive cardiomyopathy with a nondilated or small LV cavity [2], as in case 2. LV systolic function may be normal or reduced, and biatrial enlargement is common, reflecting the elevated filling pressure, such as in case 1. Other distinctive pictures include diffuse valvular thickening with mild regurgitation in majority of patients. Doppler evaluation of transmitral and pulmonary vein, blood flow velocity shows a restrictive filling pattern. Amyloid cardiomyopathy seems to be associated with a marked dissociation between short and long-axis systolic function. Assessment of long-axis contraction using tissue Doppler or strain rate imaging shows severe impairment in long-axis contraction, even when the LV ejection fraction is within normal range [3].

References

1. Buja LM, Khol NB, Roberts WC. Clinically significant cardiac amuloidosis clinicopathologic findings in 15 patients. *Am J Cardiol* 1975;26:394.
2. Klein AL, Hatle LK, Taliercio CP, *et al.* Serial Doppler echocardiographic follow-up of LV diastolic function in cardiac amyloidosis. *J Am Coll Cardiol* 1990;16:1135.
3. Sun JP, Stewart WJ, Yang XS, *et al.* Differentiation of hypertrophic cardiomyopathy and cardiac amyloidosis from other causes of ventricular wall thickening by two-dimensional strain imaging echocardiography. *Am J Cardiol* 2009;103:411–15.

85 Apical Ballooning Syndrome

Jing Ping Sun[1], Xing Sheng Yang[1] & James D. Thomas[2]

[1]Emory University School of Medicine; Emory University Hospital Midtown, Atlanta, GA, USA
[2]The Cleveland Clinic Foundation, Cleveland, OH, USA

History

A 70-year-old female with a history of anxiety disorder was admitted to hospital because of abrupt chest pain and shortness of breath.

Physical Examination

Blood pressure was 80/45 mmHg; heart rate was 110 beats/minute. Jugular venous distension, bilateral crackles up to the midchest, and third heart sound were noted.

Laboratory

Electrocardiogram showed a typical ST-segment elevation on admission, and abnormal QS-wave in V1-3 on the second day (Figure 85.1). Echocardiogram showed extensive anteroapical akinesis with basal function preserved, which led to mitral anterior leaflet anterior movement during systole (Figure 85.2a and Videoclip 85.1) and mitral regurgitation (MR) (Figure 85.2b). The sequence of our patient's presentation suggests that the apical ballooning caused geometric alterations of left ventricle (LV) that in turn led to acute MR, systolic anterior motion, and mid LV obstruction (Figure 85.2c, Videoclip 85.2). Right ventricle systolic function was normal.

Coronary angiography demonstrated nonobstructive coronary disease.

Practical Handbook of Echocardiography 1st edition. Edited by Jing Ping Sun, Joel Felner and John Merlino. © 2010 Blackwell Publishing Ltd.

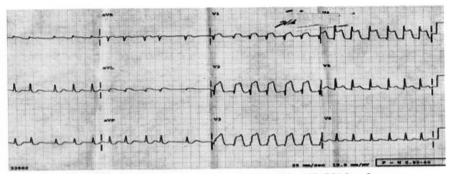

EKG day 1: ST segment elevated in V2-V4 leads

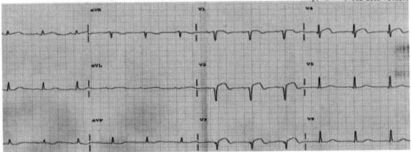

EKG day 2: Elevted ST segment recovered to baseline

Figure 85.1. Electrocardiogram showed a typical ST-segment elevation on admission and abnormal QS-wave in V1-3 on the second day.

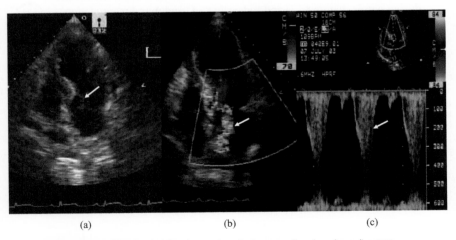

(a)   (b)   (c)

Figure 85.2. Apical 4-chamber view and continuous wave Doppler echocardiograms revealing extensive anteroapical akinesis and the basal function preserved, which lead to mitral anterior leaflet anterior movement during systole (a, arrow) and mitral regurgitation (b, arrow). The sequence of our patient's presentation suggests that the apical ballooning caused geometric alterations of LV that in turn led to acute mitral regurgitation, systolic anterior motion, and mid left ventricular obstruction (c, high velocity).

Discussion

The apical ballooning syndrome (ABS) is also called Takotsubo cardiomyopathy. The precise incidence of ABS is unknown. Review of the literature reported a prevalence of 1.7–2.2% of patients presenting with acute coronary syndrome [1].

The most common presenting clinical symptoms were chest pain, dyspnea, and simulation of acute myocardial infarction. The most common abnormalities were ST-segment elevation and T wave inversion, usually observed during the acute and subacute phases. Coronary arteriography shows no critical lesions [2]

Usually, patients had marked LV apical dysfunction on admission, mean EF ranging from 20 to 49% [1]. A transient, dynamic intraventricular pressure gradient was found in some cases in the literature [1]. During the acute phase, all patients had moderate-to-severe midventricular dysfunction and apical akinesis or dyskinesis with the basal function preserved or hyperkinetic. However, over a period of days to weeks, all patients experienced a dramatic improvement or completely resolved their LV function. The onset of stress-induced cardiomyopathy is typically triggered by an acute medical illness or by intense emotional or physical stress. The pathophysiology of ABS is not well understood.

Clinicians should prudently consider this syndrome in the differential diagnoses of chest pain and dyspnea, especially in postmenopausal women with a recent history of emotional, physical, or medical stress.

References
1. Gianni M, Dentali F, Grandi AM, *et al.* Apical ballooning syndrome or takotsubo cardiomyopathy: a systematic review. *Eur Heart J* 2006;27:1523–9.
2. Tsuchihashi K, Ueshima K, Uchida T, *et al.* Transient apical ballooning without coronary artery stenosis: a novel heart syndrome mimicking acute myocardial infarction. Angina pectoris – myocardial infarction investigators in Japan. *J Am Coll Cardiol* 2001;38:11–18.

86 Noncompaction Cardiomyopathy

Xing Sheng Yang & Jing Ping Sun

Emory University School of Medicine; Emory University Hospital Midtown, Atlanta, GA, USA

History

A 50-year-old female complains of chest pain. She has a known history of nonischemic cardiomyopathy with an ejection fraction of 20%, status post implantable cardioverter defibrillator placement with a biventricular pacemaker, and a history of atrial fibrillation with rapid ventricular rhythm.

Physical Examination

Temperature was 35.6°C, respiration rate was 22/minute, pulse rate was 102/minute, and blood pressure was 77/44 mmHg. Cardiovascular exam showed an irregular rate. No murmurs, rubs, or gallops were heard.

Laboratory

Echocardiogram: The ventricular size is moderately dilated with severe hypertrophy, and systolic function is severely decreased. Inferoseptal wall from mid-ventricle to base is severely hypokinetic. The pattern of left ventricular hypertrophy is strongly suggestive of noncompaction (Figure 86.1, Videoclip 86.1). A maximal end systolic ratio of noncompacted to compacted layers was >2. There were mild to moderate aortic and mitral valvular regurgitations. Left atrium was severely dilated.

Magnetic resonance imaging revealed deep trabeculations in the ventricular wall, which define recesses communicating with the main ventricular chamber (Videoclip 86.2). The ratio of maximal thickness of the noncompacted to compacted layers (measured at end diastole in a parasternal short-axis view) was >2.

Practical Handbook of Echocardiography 1st edition. Edited by Jing Ping Sun, Joel Felner and John Merlino. © 2010 Blackwell Publishing Ltd.

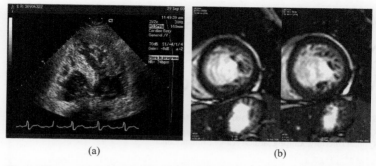

(a)   (b)

Figure 86.1. Apical 4-chamber view demonstrates deep trabeculations in left ventricular and right ventricular wall (a). Magnetic resonance images (b) show deep trabeculations in left ventricular and right ventricular wall trabeculations with maximal diastolic ratio of noncompaction to compacted thickness of >2.0.

Discussion

Noncompaction cardiomyopathy is a rare congenital cardiomyopathy that affects both children and adults and refers to a type of cardiomyopathy where the myocardial development is hindered while the fetus is in utero during the embryogenesis stage.

Noncompaction cardiomyopathy is characterized anatomically by deep trabeculations in the ventricular wall, which define recesses communicating with the main ventricular chamber. Three major clinical manifestations of noncompaction have been described: heart failure, arrhythmias, and embolic events.

Echocardiography has been the diagnostic test of choice for noncompaction. Other modalities have been used for the diagnosis, including contrast ventriculography, computed tomography, and MRI.

Treatment for noncompaction of the ventricular myocardium focuses on the three major clinical manifestations. Cardiac transplantation has been used for those with refractory congestive heart failure only.

87 A Rare Case of Isolated Noncompaction of the Right Ventricular Myocardium

Guang Zhi[1], Xiao Juan Zhang[1], LuYue Gai[1] & Patrick E. BeDell[2]
[1]General Hospital of PLA, Beijing, China
[2]Clinical Directory, Xinjiang Medical School Urumqi, China

History

A 23-year-old female presented with a 5-month history of bilateral lower extremity edema and exertional shortness of breath.

Physical Examination

Blood pressure was 120/80 mmHg, heart rate was regular at 76 bpm, respiratory rate was 18/minute, and temperature was 36.3°C. Cardiac auscultation revealed a normal first and second heart sound. A systolic murmur was heard at the third intercostal space.

Laboratory

Chest X-ray revealed large bilateral pleural effusions.

Transthoracic echocardiography (TTE): left ventricle (LV) and left atrium were normal in size and in systolic function. Right ventricle (RV) was mildly dilated; right atrium was significantly dilated. Trabeculation with deep fissures and grooves were noted in the RV apical wall (Figure 87.1). Mild tricuspid regurgitation was noted with maximum velocity of 0.47 m/sec. The forward flow velocity through the pulmonary valve was reduced with a maximum velocity of 0.45 m/sec. The RV global contraction was hypokinetic. RV apical region displayed a sponge-like appearance, characteristic of noncompacted myocardium (Figure 87.2a).

The magnetic resonance images are shown in Figure 87.2.

Management

Based on the test results and clinical manifestation, a diagnosis of RV noncompaction was made. Diuretics were administered in order to relieve the patient's right heart failure.

Practical Handbook of Echocardiography 1st edition. Edited by Jing Ping Sun, Joel Felner and John Merlino. © 2010 Blackwell Publishing Ltd.

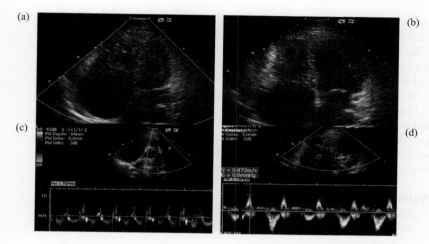

Figure 87.1. Apical 4-chamber view shows the typical pattern of noncompaction with prominent trabeculations in the apical of right ventricle. Color Doppler flow mapping demonstrates flow between the sinusoids (a). No noncompaction of the left ventricle is noted (b); pulse wave Doppler recording demonstrates forward blood flow of pulmonary artery (c) and tricuspid valve regurgitation; (d) velocities from both are significantly reduced.

Discussion

Isolated noncompaction of the ventricular myocardium (NCVM) is a rare congenital anomaly characterized by multiple myocardial sinusoids [1, 2].

LV noncompaction was first described more than a decade ago and is usually associated with the development of abnormal LV function [1,3]. Cases of isolated ventricular noncompaction involving only RV were not reported until recently. In our case, the clinical symptoms and CMR

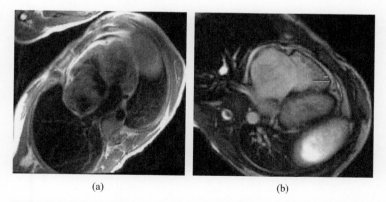

(a)   (b)

Figure 87.2. Magnetic resonance images revealed (a) FSE black blood sequence images show no fat suppression. (b) Sequence images show the right ventricle apical trabeculations with maximal diastolic ratio of noncompaction (red tracing) to compacted thickness (green tracing) of >3.0.

excluded the diagnosis of arrhythmogenic RV cardiomyopathy. TTE demonstrated numerous marked sinusoids in the region of the RV apical wall and normal morphology and position of the tricuspid valve. Based on the findings of the cardiac magnetic resonance imaging, TTE, right heart catheterization, and ventriculogram, the patient's diagnosis is reasonably clear: isolated noncompaction of RV myocardium.

With the use of diagnostic imaging techniques on the rise, in the future, isolated noncompaction of RV may be found to have an increasing prevalence in the general population. The long-term outlook for this asymptomatic cohort of patients with isolated RV noncompaction is still unclear, but may not be as sinister as first thought.

References

1. Chin TK, Perloff JK, Williams RG, Jue K, Mohrmann R. Isolated non-compaction of left ventricular myocardium. A study of eight cases. *Circulation* 1990;82:507–13.
2. Karatza A, Holder RSE, Gardiner H.M. Isolated non-compaction of the ventricular myocardium: prenatal diagnosis and natural history. *Ultrasound Obstet Gynecol* 2003;21:75–80.
3. Duncan RF, Brown MA, Worthley SG, *et al.* Increasing identification of isolated left ventricular non-compaction with cardiovascular magnetic resonance: a mini case series highlighting variable clinical presentation. *Heart Lung Circ* 2008;17:9–13.

Part 11
Miscellaneous

88 Role of Echocardiography in Cardiac Resynchronization Therapy

Jing Ping Sun & Xing Sheng Yang
Emory University School of Medicine; Emory University Hospital Midtown, Atlanta, GA, USA

Medical therapy has led to marked improvements in both symptom control and overall survival in patients with heart failure (HF). Implanted devices, such as implantable cardioverter defibrillators (ICDs) and pacemakers, are also beneficial. ICDs are now recommended for primary prevention of sudden cardiac death in selected patients. Some patients benefit from simultaneously pacing both ventricles, such as those with left bundle branch block. This approach is referred to as cardiac resynchronization therapy (CRT). The rationale for CRT is that ventricular dyssynchrony can further impair the pump function of a failing ventricle. Resynchronization may improve pump performance and reverse ventricular remodeling.

We present a patient with dilated cardiomyopathy and heart failure. His left ventricular ejection fraction (LV EF) was 25%. After implantation of biventricular pacing device, left ventricle (LV) contraction was significantly better when BiV pacing turned on than when it was off, which demonstrated by real-time two-dimensional images (Videoclip 88.1). Six months later, his LV EF increased to 45%, and the diastolic dysfunction improved from stage III (restrictive) to stage II (relaxation impaired). (Figure 88.1).

The benefit of CRT was illustrated in a meta-analysis of 14 randomized, controlled trials that included 4420 patients [1]. The following benefits of CRT were noted: (1) greater likelihood of improving at least one NYHA class; (2) improvements in the 6-minute walk distance and quality of life; (3) reduced rate of hospitalization for HF; and (4) reduction in all-cause mortality due to fewer deaths from progressive heart failure.

The indications for CRT are (1) patients with LV ejection fractions ≤35%; (2) a QRS duration ≥120 ms; and (3) NYHA functional class III or ambulatory class IV symptoms with optimal medical therapy [2].

Numerous single-center studies reported that improvement of LV function after CRT can be predicted by echocardiographic parameters in patients with HF. A multicenter, prospective, nonrandomized PROSPECT study of 498 patients with standard CRT indications found that 12 echocardiographic dyssynchrony parameters (including seven TDI parameters) resulted in only modest sensitivity and specificity in the ability

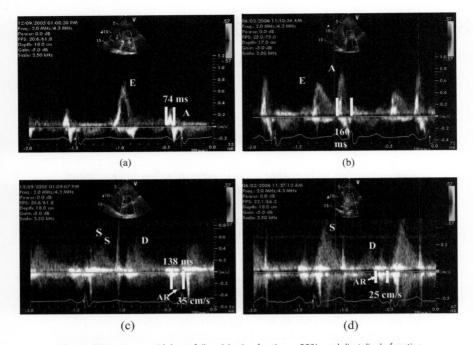

Figure 88.1. A case with heart failure (ejection fraction = 25%, and diastolic dysfunction stage III) (a and c) before cardiac resynchronization therapy (CRT); 6 months after CRT, his left ventricular ejection fraction improved to 45% and diastolic dysfunction to stage II (b and d). AR, atrial reversal

to predict clinical composite score response [3]. For all parameters, the area under the receiver–operator characteristics curve for clinical or volume response to CRT was ≤0.62. In addition, there was large variability in the analysis of the dyssynchrony parameters. Therefore, no ideal approach has been found to improve patient selection for CRT.

In summary, the role of echocardiography are (1) to select the patients according to guidelines before CRT; (2) to screen for atrioventricular optimization using Doppler mitral inflow velocities post CRT; and (3) to estimate cardiac function and remodeling for follow-up.

References

1. McAlister FA, Ezekowitz J, Hooton N, *et al.* Cardiac resynchronization therapy for patients with left ventricular systolic dysfunction: a systematic review. *JAMA* 2007;297:2502.
2. Epstein AE, DiMarco JP, Ellenbogen KA, *et al.* ACC/AHA/HRS Guidelines for device-based therapy of cardiac rhythm abnormalities: a report of the American College of Cardiology/American Heart Association Task Force on Practice Guidelines developed in collaboration with the American Association for Thoracic Surgery and Society of Thoracic Surgeons. *Circulation* 2008;117:e350.
3. Chung ES, Leon AR, Tavazzi L, *et al.* Results of the predictors of response to CRT (PROSPECT) trial. *Circulation* 2008;117:2608.

89 Cardiac Tamponade Caused by Penetrating Atheromatous Ulcer and Intramural Hematoma Involving Ascending Aorta

Ming-Jui Hung[1] & Jing Ping Sun[2]

[1] Chang Gung University College of Medicine; Chang Gung Memorial Hospital at Keelung, Keelung, Taiwan.

[2] Emory University School of Medicine; Emory University Hospital Midtown, Atlanta, GA, USA

Case History

A 70-year-old female was admitted with sudden onset of severe chest pain and dyspnea.

Physical Examination

Temperature was 36.2°C, pulse rate was 112/minute, respiration rate was 21/minute, and blood pressure was 87/59 mmHg. Her jugular vein was engorged, with an estimated right atrial pressure of more than 15 cm H_2O. The cardiac examination revealed tachycardia with a regular rhythm and no murmurs or gallops.

Laboratory

Chest X-ray revealed cardiomegaly and widening of the mediastinum.

The transthoracic echocardiography (TTE) suggested a large pericardial effusion with cardiac tamponade (Figure 89.1, Videoclip 89.1). Penetrating atheromatous ulcer and intramural hematoma in the ascending aorta were detected by computed tomography (Figure 89.2).

Practical Handbook of Echocardiography 1st edition. Edited by Jing Ping Sun, Joel Felner and John Merlino. © 2010 Blackwell Publishing Ltd.

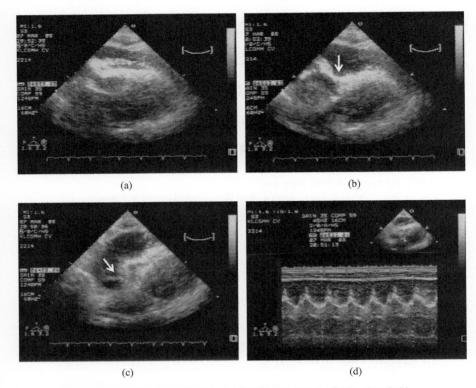

(a)

(b)

(c)

(d)

Figure 89.1. Subcostal view shows pericardial effusion containing floating thrombi (a) complicated by right ventricle (b, arrow) and right atrium (c, arrow) tamponade and confirmed by M-mode echocardiography of right ventricle end-diastolic collapse (d).

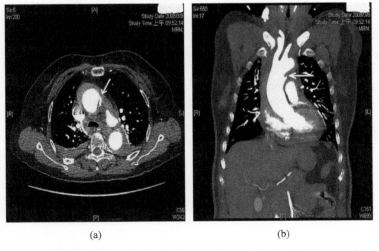

(a)

(b)

Figure 89.2. Penetrating atheromatous ulcer and intramural hematoma in the ascending aorta (a and b, arrows).

Management

She was operated on the second day after admission and monitored uneventfully for 6 months after surgery.

Discussion

Acute aortic syndrome describes the acute presentation of patients with one of several life-threatening thoracic aortic pathologies. These include aortic dissection, intramural hematoma, and penetrating atheromatous ulcer (PAU). These conditions are characterized clinically by severely intense, acute, tearing, throbbing, and migratory chest pain in patients with coexisting history of hypertension. Occasionally some patients exhibited some or all of these lesions as did our patient, demonstrating the link between these pathologies. The clinical progress of these patients is unpredictable, and an early diagnosis is essential. Our patient had a history of hypertension and also complained of sudden onset of severe chest pain associated with syncope, which were consistent with acute aortic syndrome, without evidence of acute myocardial injury.

The differential diagnosis in this situation includes acute coronary syndrome, aortic dissection, intramural hematoma, true aneurysm, and pulmonary embolism. Anterior chest pain tends to correlate with ascending aortic lesions as in our patient, while descending aortic lesions usually cause back pain [1]. With PAU, there is a paucity of specific clinical signs, for example, there is no pulse deficit, aortic regurgitation, stroke, or visceral compromise [2]. The risk of aortic rupture is significantly higher in patients with PAU [1]. Early intervention is indicated if there are signs suggestive of aortic disease progression.

Our patient was diagnosed with a ruptured PAU and intramural hematoma involving the ascending aorta complicated by cardiac tamponade and pleural effusion within 24 hours after admission. Cardiac tamponade was demonstrated by TTE; pericardiocentesis was performed under TTE guiding. Urgent operation was successfully performed.

References

1. Coady MA, Rizzo JA, Elefteriades JA. Pathologic variants of thoracic aortic dissections. Penetrating atherosclerotic ulcers and intramural hematomas. *Cardiol Clin* 1999;17:637–57.
2. Cooke JP, Kazmier FJ, Orszulak TA. The penetrating aortic ulcer: pathologic manifestations, diagnosis, and management. *Mayo Clin Proc* 1988;63:718–25.

90 Iatrogenic Dissection of Coronary Sinus Secondary to Angioplasty

Jing Ping Sun[1] & Joel M. Felner[2]

[1] Emory University School of Medicine; Emory University Hospital Midtown, Atlanta, GA, USA
[2] Grady Memorial Hospital; Emory University School of Medicine, Atlanta, GA, USA

History and Physical Examination

A 70-year-old man was admitted with persistent chest pain. He was a smoker and was diagnosed with hypertension for 10 years. A physical examination was unremarkable.

Laboratory and Hospital Course

Electrocardiogram showed ST segment elevation in leads II, III, and aVF.

ST depression with inverted T wave was found in leads I, aVL, V4, and V5.

Blood chemistry tests revealed the elevation of cardiac enzymes. He was diagnosed with acute inferior myocardial infarction and underwent emergency coronary angiography. Selected coronary angiography demonstrated total occlusion in the proximal portion of right coronary artery (RCA). Left ventriculography showed akinesis of the inferior wall with an ejection fraction of 55%. Percutaneous coronary intervention (PCI) was immediately performed for the culprit lesion of the RCA. When a guiding catheter and BMW guidewire were inserted into the right coronary sinus, but met resistant. Transesophageal echocardiography (TEE) was performed and found localized injury in the aortic root (right coronary sinus) and causing a small dissection (Figures 90.1, 90.2 and Videoclip 90.1). Although he had no specific complaints and his vital signs did not change, the procedure was postponed. He was treated conservatively without any anticoagulants or antiplatelet medicines, and his systolic blood pressure was controlled under 130 mmHg. Thereafter, his clinical course was uneventful without any complications.

Transthoracic echocardiography performed just after the accident and after 18 days showed neither aortic regurgitation nor dissection in the aortic root. PCI was successfully performed at the same day. Before the PCI, complete resolution of the dissection in the right coronary sinus was confirmed angiographically. Patient did well during a 8-month follow-up.

Practical Handbook of Echocardiography 1st edition. Edited by Jing Ping Sun, Joel Felner and John Merlino. © 2010 Blackwell Publishing Ltd.

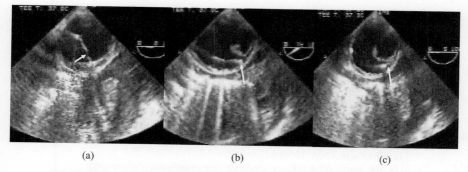

(a)   (b)   (c)

Figure 90.1. Transesophageal echocardiogram sequence of aortic short-axis views illustrate (arrows) a catheter-tip injury causing an aortic root dissection (a–c).

Discussion

Localized dissection of the sinus of Valsalva is an extremely rare accident that may occur during percutaneous coronary intervention, but it can lead to serious complications such as dissection of the ascending aorta. Although dissection of the sinus of Valsalva and aortic wall following coronary artery dissection induced by a guiding catheter or guidewire has been previously reported [1], a localized dissection of the coronary cusp without coronary artery involvement has not yet been reported as we know.

Iatrogenic coronary artery dissection involving the adjacent aortic wall has been treated successfully with conservative treatment, stenting, and surgery [2, 3]. Perez-Castellano et al. have reported that the localized dissections of the sinus of Valsalva tend to resolve spontaneously within a month because of the particular anatomy of the sinus of Valsalva. In our case, a catheter-tip injury causing a small aortic root

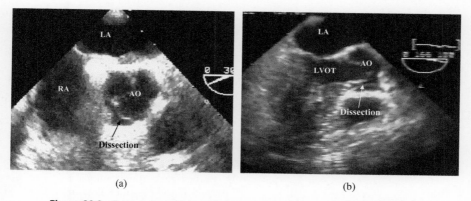

(a)   (b)

Figure 90.2. Transesophageal echocardiogram aortic short-axis view illustrates a dissection in the aortic root (a). Transesophageal echocardiogram long-axis view shows the dissection (b). AO, aorta; LA, left atrium; LVOT, left ventricular outflow tract; RA, right atrium.

dissection, which was detected by TEE immediately. PCI was postponed and successfully performed 18 days later; the patient recovered well.

References

1. Perez-Castellano N, Garcia-Fernandez MA, Garcia EJ, Delcan JL. Dissection of the aortic sinus of Valsalva complicating coronary catheterization: cause, mechanism, evolution, and management. *Cathet Cardiovasc Diagn* 1998;43:273–9.
2. Goldstein JA, Casserly IP, Katsiyiannis WT, Lasala JM, Taniuchi M. Aortocoronary dissection complicating a percutaneous coronary intervention. *J Invasive Cardiol* 2003;15:89–92 (review).
3. Vega MR. Aortic dissection – exceedingly rare complication of coronary angioplasty. *Cathet Cardiovasc Diagn* 1997;42:416.

91 Hypereosinophilic Syndromes

Jing Ping Sun[1], Xing Sheng Yang[1] & Joel M. Felner[2]

[1]Emory University School of Medicine; Emory University Hospital Midtown, Atlanta, GA, USA
[2]Grady Memorial Hospital, Emory University School of Medicine, Atlanta, GA, USA

History

A 60-year-old male complains of onset of weakness, malaise, and dyspnea on exertion. He has a history of chronic kidney disease and hypertension. He has no known drug allergies.

Physical Examination

Blood pressure was 104/82 mmHg, heart rate was 106 and regular, respiration rate was 26/minute, and temperature was 37°C. Precordial movements—apex impulse was slightly displaced laterally.

Laboratory

Chest X-ray revealed diffuse, hazy infiltrates bilaterally. Complete blood count was remarkable for elevated eosinophil count of 59% with a total white blood cell count of 10.3.

Electrocardiogram results: normal sinus rhythm, low voltage and nonspecific ST-T wave changes.

Endomyocardial biopsy: acute myocarditis, diffuse, with mixed inflammatory cells and numerous eosinophils consistent with Loeffler's myocarditis. Magnetic resonance imaging (MRI) of brain revealed multiple cerebral infarcts, suggestive of an embolic source.

Echocardiography

Left ventricle (LV) is normal in size and function with mild left ventricular hypertrophy. There are two mobile masses attached to the midinferior wall in apical 2-chamber view and three mobile structures on the septum in A4-ch view (Figure 91.1 and Videoclip 91.1,91.2). There is diastolic dysfunction consistent with impaired relaxation. The right side of heart and cardiac valve are normal in structures and function. The second study was done after treatment. The previously noted mobile mass on the ventricular septum is no longer seen (Videoclip 96.2).

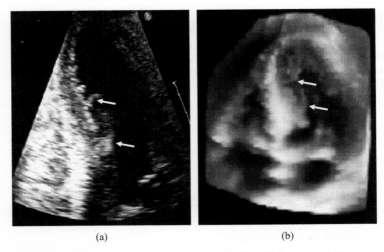

(a)   (b)

Figure 91.1. There are two mobile masses attached to the midinferior wall (a). There are two mobile structures on the septum (b) in case 1.

For presentation, a case with right ventricle (RV) apical thrombus is shown in Figure 91.2 and Videoclip 96.3.

Hospital Course

Case 1: The patient was treated with steroids and his eosinophil count responded briskly.

After treatment, a repeat echocardiogram done showed that the previously seen LV thrombus disappeared. Follow-up was done for 6 years; the patient was doing well.

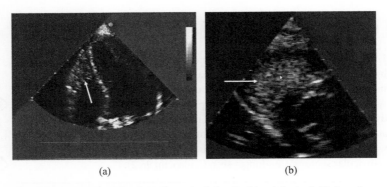

(a)   (b)

Figure 91.2. Transthoracic echocardiography 4-chamber (a) and short-axis (b) views show right ventricular thrombus (arrow) in case 2.

Discussion

The associations among eosinophilia, active carditis, and multiorgan involvement were first described by Loeffler in 1936 [1]. Pathologic specimens in Loeffler endocarditis show eosinophilic myocarditis, a tendency toward endomyocardial fibrosis and clinical manifestations of thromboembolism, and acute heart failure.

Eosinophil-mediated heart damage evolves through three stages [1]: (1) an acute necrotic stage; (2) an intermediate phase characterized by thrombus formation along the damaged endocardium; and (3) a fibrotic stage. Our case was suffered with acute myocarditis belong to first stage; this stage responded to steroids therapy briskly.

In the face of a non-dilated, hypokinetic LV and RV with biventricular apical thrombi and hypereosinophilia should raise the clinical suspicion of the idiopathic hypereosinophilic syndrome.

Echocardiography may demonstrate intracardiac thrombi and evidence of fibrosis, such as thickening of the posterior mitral valve leaflet or the posterior wall, and increases in endomyocardial echodensity in areas of fibrosis. MRI reliably detects all stages and aspects of eosinophil-mediated heart damage, including the early stage of myocardial eosinophilic inflammation.

Reference

1. Loeffler W. Endocarditis parietalis fibroplastica mit Blut-eosinophilie, ein eigenartiges Krankheitshild. *Schweiz Med Wochenschr* 1936;66:817–20.

92 Echocardiographic Evaluation of the Atria and Appendages

Jing Ping Sun & John D. Merlino

Emory University School of Medicine; Emory University Hospital Midtown, Atlanta, GA, USA

History

A 60-year-old male presented with a history of stroke and rheumatic fever as a child.

Physical Examination

The blood pressure was 131/75 mmHg, the heart rate was 108/minute, and the respiration rate was 20/minute.

Cardiovascular examination: He was in irregularly rhythm. There was a diastolic murmur at the apex. Neck veins were normal.

Laboratory

An electrocardiogram revealed atrial fibrillation.

Echocardiography: Transthoracic echocardiography (TTE) revealed normal left ventricle (LV) size, structure, and wall thickness with normal systolic function. Left atrial cavity size is severely dilated. Mitral valve: There is typical mitral leaflet moderately thickening and commisural fusion, consistent with moderate rheumatic mitral valve stenosis (Figure 92.1). A mass can be seen in left atrium (LA), which is not clear (Figure 92.2a and Videoclip 92.1a). A mild degree of mitral regurgitation is seen by color Doppler. The aortic valve is tricuspid with trace aortic regurgitation.

Transesophageal echocardiography (TEE): Large thrombi were seen in LA appendage and LA. Some were mobile (Figure 92.2b and c and 92.2 b–d). There is no evidence of patent foramen ovale.

Practical Handbook of Echocardiography 1st edition. Edited by Jing Ping Sun, Joel Felner and John Merlino. © 2010 Blackwell Publishing Ltd.

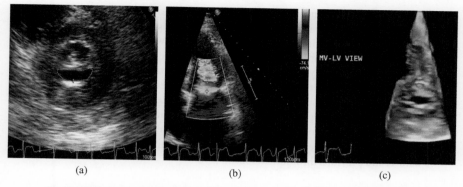

(a)   (b)   (c)

Figure 92.1. Parasternal short-axis view shows the mitral leaflets are thickened, and the opening of mitral valvular orifice is small (a). Apical 4-chamber view shows the high-velocity inflow through the narrow mitral orifice by color Doppler (b). Three-dimensional echocardiography shows the thickened mitral leaflets and the small orifice of mitral valve (c). All of the signs above are consistent with rheumatic mitral stenosis. LV, left ventricle; MV, mitral valve.

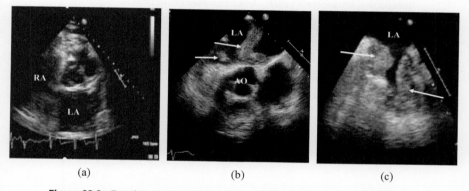

(a)   (b)   (c)

Figure 92.2. Transthoracic echocardiography: It is hard to see the thrombus in left atrium from parasternal short-axis view (a). Transesophageal echocardiography: Several thrombi are well seen in left atrium (b); the thrombus filling in the left atrial appendage (c). AO, aorta; LA, left atrium; RA, right atrium.

Discussion

The LA appendage is a common site for atrial thrombi and may be the cause of cardiogenic thromboembolism [1]. In patients with a stroke and/or atrial fibrillation, it is important to rule out the presence of left atrial appendage thrombi.

TEE permits examination of most of LA, including excellent views of LA appendage; it is the preferred approach for the detection of thrombi in LA and appendage, being much more sensitive than TTE [2]. Left atrial thrombi are often multiple and vary in size and, although they attach to the atrial wall, they usually demonstrate some degree of independent motion.

The finding of spontaneous echo contrast, indicative of predisposing stasis, almost always accompanies thrombus and may be helpful in differentiating thrombi from tumor. In our case, the thrombi in LA was hard to see in TTE image, but the thrombi and spontaneous echo contrast in LA and appendage were clearly demonstrated by TEE. Patients with persistent atrial fibrillation undergoing cardioversion are frequently anticoagulated with *warfarin* for at least three to four weeks in an attempt to permit resolution of possible preexisting thrombi. In such patients, routine TEE before cardioversion following prolonged anticoagulation is not routinely recommended but can be considered in those with mitral stenosis, heart failure, and previous thromboembolism.

References

1. Jordan RA, Scheifley CH, Edwards JE. Mural thrombosis and arterial embolism in mitral stenosis. A clinicopathologic study of fifty-one cases. *Circulation* 1951;3:363–7.
2. Manning WJ, Weintraub RM, Waksmonski CA, *et al.* Accuracy of transesophageal echocardiography for identifying left atrial thrombi. A prospective, intraoperative study. *Ann Intern Med* 1995;123:817.

93 Lipomatous Hypertrophy of the Interatrial Septum

Xing Sheng Yang, Jing Ping Sun & John D. Merlino
Emory University School of Medicine; Emory University Hospital Midtown, Atlanta, GA, USA

History

A 80-year-old female has a history of cardiac bypass with no symptom.

Physical Examination

She was overweight. Cardiac examination was unremarkable except for a mild systolic murmur.

Laboratory Study

Transthoracic echocardiography showed an intracardiac atrial septal lesion and that the probable diagnosis was lipomatous hypertrophy of the interatrial septum. Transesophageal echocardiography: Lipomatous hypertrophy of the interatrial septum appears as a bilobar echogenic enlargement of the interatrial septum sparing the fossa ovalis (Figure 93.1 and Videoclip 93.1).

Discussion

Lipomatous hypertrophy of the interatrial septum is not uncommon now and is increasingly recognized with the use of echocardiography, computed tomography, and magnetic resonance imaging. It was first described by Prior [1] in 1964 in five patients at a postmortem examination.

Lipomatous hypertrophy is due to a proliferation of fat cells rather than hypertrophy of the cells and consists of an unencapsulated accumulation of mature adipose tissue with cells resembling brown fat. It is more common in the old age and in those with obesity.

In echocardiography, lipomatous hypertrophy of the interatrial septum appears as a bilobar echogenic enlargement of the interatrial septum

Practical Handbook of Echocardiography 1st edition. Edited by Jing Ping Sun, Joel Felner and John Merlino. © 2010 Blackwell Publishing Ltd.

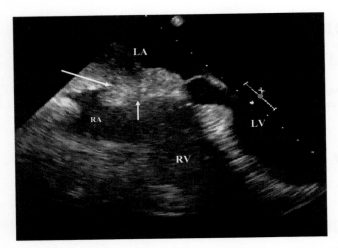

Figure 93.1. Lipomatous hypertrophy of the interatrial septum appears as a bilobar echogenic enlargement of the interatrial septum (arrow) sparing the fossa ovalis (small arrow). LA, left atrium; LV, left ventricle; RA, right atrium; RV, right ventricle.

sparing the fossa ovalis, dumbbell-shaped mass of fat attenuation with smooth margins. The masses can generally be distinguished from pathologic masses by the absence of involvement of the fossa ovalis.

Lipomatous hypertrophy requires no further cardiac workup or therapy.

References

1. Prior JT. Lipomatous hypertrophy of cardiac interatrial septum. *Arch Pathol* 1964;78:11–15.

94 Apicoaortic Bypass

Jing Ping Sun, Alicia N. Rangosch, Robert D. O'Donnell Jr., Dan Sorescu & John D. Merlino

Emory University School of Medicine; Emory University Hospital Midtown, Atlanta, GA, USA

History

A 60-year-old male has an apicoaortic conduit placed 1 month ago for critical aortic stenosis.

Physical Examination

Heart: regular rate and rhythm, no extra heart sounds, no murmurs.
   Lungs: clear.

Echocardiography

The preoperative echo demonstrates severe aortic valve stenosis with an aortic valve area of 0.6 cm² (Figure 94.1). The ascending aorta was heavily calcified. This was felt to preclude a standard aortic valve replacement surgery. The postapicoaortic placement, transthoracic echocardiography (TTE): (a) Parasternal long-axis view reveals a conduit below left ventricle (LV) posterior wall entering descending aorta. (b) parasternal short axis

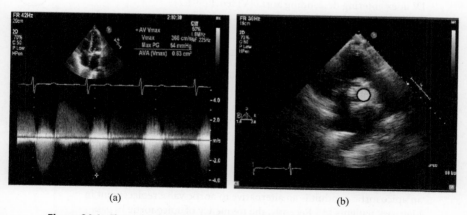

(a)   (b)

Figure 94.1. The peak velocity of aortic flow was 3.7 m/sec, maximal gradient = 54 mmHg (a). The area of aortic orifice was 0.62 cm² (b).

Practical Handbook of Echocardiography 1st edition. Edited by Jing Ping Sun, Joel Felner and John Merlino. © 2010 Blackwell Publishing Ltd.

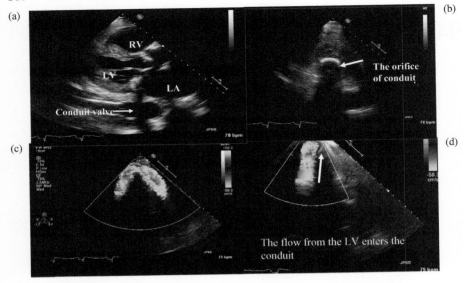

Figure 94.2. Parasternal long-axis view reveals a conduit below left ventricular posterior wall entering descending aorta (a). PAS view shows the orifice of conduit in apex (b). Apical view shows the conduit from the apex along left ventricular lateral wall (c). Apical view shows the flow entering conduit (d). LA, left atrium; LV, left ventricle; RV, right ventricle.

view shows the orifice of conduit in apex. (c) Apical view shows the conduit from the apex, along the lateral LV wall. (d) Apical view shows the flow entering conduit (Figure 94.2). The valve of conduit is functioning well (Videoclip 94.1, 2)

Magnetic resonance imaging reveals the entire apicoaortic conduit from LV apex entering descending aorta (Videoclip 94.2).

Discussion

In 1977, Reder *et al.* reported a case in which a 17-year-old girl had operative relief of her congenital tunnel subaortic stenosis by using a valve-bearing conduit between LV apex and thoracic aorta [1]. In 1987, Tanaka reported another apicoaortic bypass operation in a patient with a calcified ascending aorta due to Werner's syndrome [2]. In cases of severely calcified ascending aortas, modified operative strategies are required in order to avoid manipulations of the aorta and hopefully to minimize the chance of subsequent cerebral vascular accidents. Aortic valve bypass with an apicoaortic conduit is an alternative to aortic valve replacement in high-risk patients [3]. Recently, the frequency of apicoaortic bypass operation has increased. Echocardiography is ease of use, low cost, and a convenient method to assess apicoaortic conduits. In our case, TTE with color Doppler demonstrated that the conduit was patent, and the valve in the conduit was functioning well.

References

1. Bonow RO, Carabello BA, Chatterjee K, *et al.* ACC/AHA Guidelines for the management of patients with valvular heart disease: executive summary *Circulation* 2006;114;450–527.
2. Reder RF, Dimich I, Steinfeld L, Litwak RS. Left ventricle to aorta valved conduit for relief of diffuse left ventricular outflow tract obstruction. *Am J Cardiol* 1977 June;39(7):1068–72.
3. Tanaka S, Kakihata H, Urayama K, Kuji N, Maida K. Apico-aortic bypass operation in a patient with calcified ascending aorta due to Werner's syndrome. *J Cardiovasc Surg (Torino)* 1987 July–August;28(4):391–4.

95 Paradoxical Strokes

Jing Ping Sun[1], Xing Sheng Yang[1] & James D. Thomas[2]
[1] Emory University School of Medicine; Emory University Hospital Midtown, Atlanta, GA, USA
[2] The Cleveland Clinic Foundation, Cleveland, OH, USA

History

A 40-year-old obese female presents with a 1-day history of weakness in the right upper and lower limbs.

Examination

Neurologic examinations revealed a right hemiparesis and mild motor dysphasia. Cerebral computed tomography scan, obtained after 24 and 72 hours, ruled out a hemorrhage.

Echocardiography

Transesophageal echocardiography (TEE) image showed a section of a thrombus with a long tail that was entrapped in a patent foramen oval. It floated in both atria and then settled in the left atrium (Figures 95.1 and 95.2 and Videoclip 95.1).

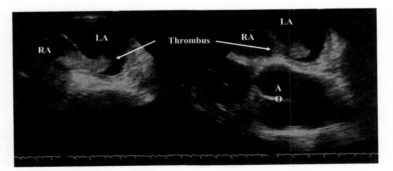

Figure 95.1. A section of this thrombus was entrapped in a patent foramen ovale and floated in both atria (left), a thrombus is dropping into left atrium (right). AO, aorta; LA, left atrium; RA, right atrium.

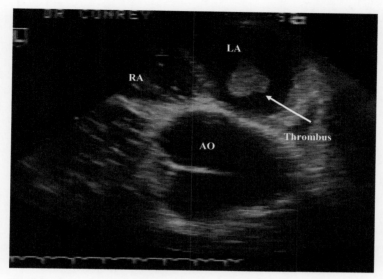

Figure 95.2. A thrombus settled in left atrium through patent foramen ovale. AO, aorta; LA, left atrium; RA, right atrium.

Treatment: This rare situation, named impending paradoxical embolism, prompted us to perform a surgical intervention, removing the thrombus and repairing the patent foramen ovale (PFO).

Discussion

It is estimated that 70,000–100,000 strokes per year in the United States are secondary to paradoxical embolism via a PFO [1]. The frequency of PFO detection with TEE in stroke patients may be as high as 40–45% [2]. A meta-analysis of several studies documented that the relative risk of stroke compared to nonstroke controls increased by a factor of 1.83 if a PFO was present [3].

Echocardiography is a useful tool to search the thrombus and PFO; TEE is more sensitive than transthoracic echocardiography [4].

There is a large thrombus in right atrium, which passes through the PFO into LA and causing stroke in our case. This referred to paradoxical embolism that is clearly seen on the TEE

References

1. Meier B, Lock JE. Contemporary management of patent foramen ovale. *Circulation* 2003;107:5–9.
2. Lamy C, Giannesini C, Zuber M, *et al.* Clinical and imaging findings in cryptogenic stroke patients with and without patent foramen ovale: the PFO-ASA Study. *Stroke* 2002;33:706–11.

3. Overell JR, Bone I, Lees KR. Interatrial septal abnormalities and stroke: a meta-analysis of case-control studies. *Neurology* 2000;55:1172–9.
4. Sun JP, Stewart WJ, Joseph Hanna JP, Thomas JD. Diagnosis of patent foramen ovale by contrast versus color Doppler using TEE: relation to atrial size. *Am Heart J* 1996;131:239–44.

96 Cardiac Tamponade Caused by Pleural Effusion

Jing Ping Sun[1], Joel M. Felner[2] & John D. Merlino[1]

[1]Emory University School of Medicine; Emory University Hospital Midtown, Atlanta, GA, USA
[2]Grady Memorial Hospital; Emory University School of Medicine, Atlanta, GA, USA

Case History

A 40-year-old male, who has a history of diffuse large B cell lymphoma stage IV, presented with progressively increasing shortness of breath for the past 4 weeks.

Physical Examination

He appears to be in marked respiratory distress. The blood pressure was 105/75 mmHg, heart rate was 121 bpm with regular rhythm, respiratory rate was 26 and temperature was 35.7°C. On pulmonary examination he had bilaterally decreased breath sounds and dullness to percussion. Cardiac examination: (1) neck veins were elevated to the angle of the jaw; (2) heart sounds were normal, but distant; and (3) there were no murmurs or extra heart sounds.

Laboratory

Chest X-ray revealed large bilateral pleural effusions.

The transthoracic echocardiography (TTE) apical views suggests a large pericardial effusion, right atrium (RA), and right ventricle (RV) collapse. But in the subcostal 4-chamber view, there was no pericardial effusion around RV free wall (Figure 96.1, Videoclip 96.1).

Management

Right and left chest tubes were inserted into the respective pleural spaces. Approximately 1500–1800 cc of colorless fluid was evacuated from each pleural cavity. The patient's ventilation improved dramatically, allowing us to perform TTE and transesophageal echocardiography that did not show a significant pericardial effusion. A small amount of fluid was present anterior to the RA (Figure 96.2, Videoclip 96.2).

Practical Handbook of Echocardiography 1st edition. Edited by Jing Ping Sun, Joel Felner and John Merlino. © 2010 Blackwell Publishing Ltd.

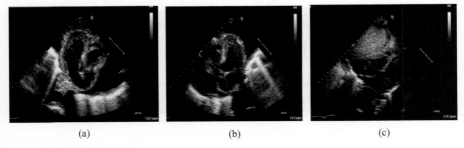

(a)   (b)   (c)

Figure 96.1. Right atrial collapse can be seen in apical views (a and b). There was no pericardial effusion around right ventricular free wall in the subcostal view (c).

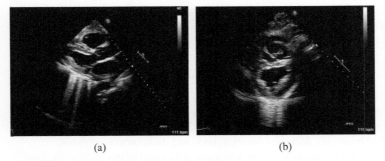

(a)   (b)

Figure 96.2. After approximately 1500–1800 cc of colorless fluid was evacuated from each pleural cavity (a and b), there was no signs of pericardial effusion.

Discussion

Pleural effusions are extremely common in critically ill patients, but their characteristics that cause hemodynamic compromise have only recently been elucidated. Vaska *et al.*'s [1] experimental results suggested that large effusions can cause increased intrapleural pressure that may be transmitted to the pericardial space. They also demonstrated, in a canine model, that RV diastolic collapse could be produced by intrapleural instillation of saline.

Cardiac tamponade caused by pleural effusions alone have only occasionally been reported, since the original description by Kisnauki *et al.* in 1991 [2]. Sadaniantz *et al.* retrospectively reviewed 116 echocardiograms from patients with pleural effusions, in the absence of a pericardial effusion, and found that 18% had RA diastolic collapse [3]. There are also other reports of RA and RV diastolic collapse without hemodynamic compromise that completely disappeared after thoracentesis for large pleural effusions.

Our case demonstrated that pleural effusions are a potential cause of cardiac tamponade. It further emphasized the importance of always performing a complete echocardiogram, including multiple views, and carefully analyzing all available images. A helpful echocardiographic sign for differentiating a pleural from a pericardial effusion is that a pericardial effusion, but not by a pleural effusion, separates the left atrium from the descending thoracic aorta. In addition, always look carefully at the subcostal view; there is no pericardial effusion surround RV free wall, which has proven to be invaluable in determining if fluid is pericardial or pleural.

References

1. Vaska K, Wann SL, Sager K, Klopfenstein HS. Pleural effusion as a cause of right ventricular diastolic collapse. *Circulation* 1992;86:609–17.
2. Kisanuki A, Shono H, Kiyonaga K, *et al.* Two-dimensional echocardiographic demonstration of left ventricular diastolic collapse due to compression by pleural effusion. *Am Heart J* 1991;122:1173–5.
3. Traylor JJ, Chan K, Wong I, Roxas JN, Chandraratna PA. Large pleural effusions producing signs of cardiac tamponade resolved by thoracentesis. *Am J Cardiol* 2002;89(1):106–8.

97 Anatomically Oriented Right and Left Ventricular Volume Measurements with Dynamic Three-Dimensional Echocardiography

Jing Ping Sun
Emory University School of Medicine; Emory University Hospital Midtown, Atlanta, GA, USA

Imaging the right ventricle is an essential and highly informative portion of the comprehensive echocardiographic evaluation. Patients with an abnormality of the left heart on echocardiographic examination often have concomitant right ventricular abnormalities.

A "teapot" configuration of right ventricle (RV) has been proposed as a model that includes the outflow tract, but this is difficult to represent mathematically. The tomographic nature of echocardiography makes it impractical to image this irregularly shaped organ in a single, encompassing plane.

A number of studies have attempted to measure the size or volume of the RV, but no method has gained wide acceptance.

Three-dimensional methods may, however, provide the flexibility required to adequately measure this structure.

More recently, rapid acquisition real-time three-dimensional (3D) echocardiography has provided an opportunity for ventricular functional and volume studies.

The newest Tomtec software provides tools for the analysis of RV and left ventricle (LV) volume and segmental and global function.

This rapid acquisition real-time3-dimensional echocardiography for the right ventricle is performed by loading full volume dataset and using the EchoPac platform and TomTech software. Three landmarks for automatic detection of the standard view planes (4-Chamber, sagittal and coronal). A standard acquisition window is used. In our case the dataset appears in the correct view and define the landmarks in specified positions. In the first short axis plane, we define the centre of the tricuspid valve and the centre of the mitral valve. Furthermore a landmark position point close to the apex in the mid of the left ventricle was set. Optionally we could define the centre of the pulmonary valve if it is visible.

This new technique is presented on figures and videoclips (Figures 97.1–97.3 and Videoclips 97.1–97.3).

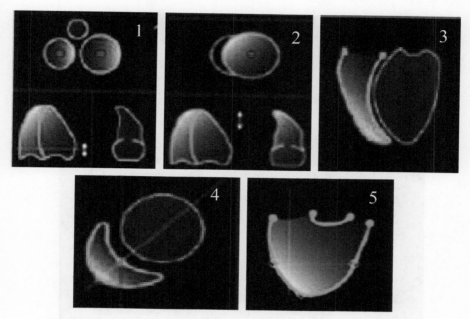

Figure 97.1.   Software technique: (1) place points in the center of the tricuspid and mitral valves as well as (2) at the center of left ventricle. Trace the right ventricular endocardium in (3) apical 4-chamber, (4) sagittal, and (5) coronal views.

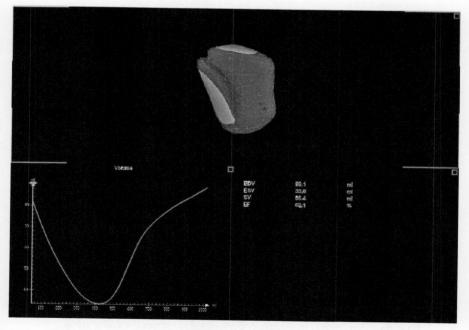

Figure 97.2.   Software results: The top panel represents the three-dimensional modeled right ventricle. The lower panel represents the time–volume curve. The end diastolic and systolic volumes are used to calculate the stroke volume and ejection fraction.

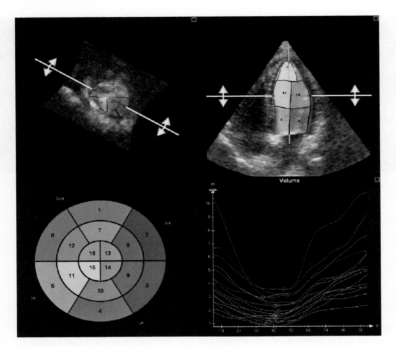

Figure 97.3. Three-dimensional echocardiography for left ventricular global and regional systolic function. The regional volume is divided in to 16-segment model (bottom left). Right lower image is the time–volume (or ejection fraction) curves (change in volume) for each individual left ventricular volume segment.

LV volume can be measured by GE 4D Auto LVQ tool (4DLVQ). This is a new volume quantification tool for rapid semi-automated detection of the LV endocardial border in real time 3D images.

This new GE 4D Auto LVQ analysis tool gives rapid and reproducible measurements of LV volumes and ejection fraction, with good agreement compared to another RT3DE volume quantication tool (Figure 97.4. and Videoclip 97.4).

When entering the tool, the user is presented with a quad-screen, showing cine loops of three apical views with 60° inter-plane spacing, and one short axis (SAX) view. If required, the apical views can be manually corrected to show the standard apical four-chamber (A4CH), apical two-chamber (A2CH), and apical long axis (ALAX) views, thereby eliminating foreshortening. When this anatomical alignment step is complete, the end-diastole (ED) frame is automatically detected from the ECG, but can be manually corrected if necessary.

While displaying the end-diastole frame, surface detection is initialized by manually selecting two points identifying the mitral annulus and one point identifying the left ventricle apex in each of the three apical views. After the total of nine landmarks are defined at end-diastole, non-temporal 3D surface detection is immediately performed to extract the endocardial border and to compute the end-diastole volume (EDV). The time required

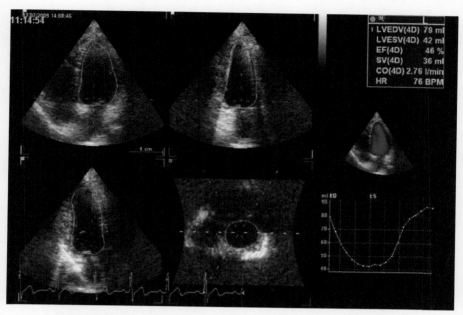

Figure 97.4. These 4 images obtained from full volume real time 3D echocardiographic data are representative 2D echocardiographic views used in the multiplanar reconstruction of the left ventricle for 3D calculation of volume and ejection automatically using GE 4D Auto LVQ tool.

for a full 3D surface detection is less than one second. Cross-sections of the detected 3D surface are displayed in three apical views and three short axis (SAX) views distributed between the LV apex and base. The above procedure is repeated for end-systole (ES). When surface detection is complete for both ED and ES, preliminary measurements of EDV, end systolic volume (ESV), and ejection fraction (EF) are presented to the user.

4D surface detection to detect LV surfaces for each frame in the entire cardiac cycle. This typically requires less than 10 seconds, depending on the frame- and heart rate, and gives a full time-volume curve. Once completed, the maximum and minimum volumes are presented on the screen as EDV and ESV respectively along with the derived EF, as shown in Figure 97.4 and Videoclips 97.4. The 3-dimensional echocardiography not only provides a tool for better assessment of left and right ventricular function, in many instances, the left and right ventricular stroke volumes can be used with the continuity equation to calculate valvular regurgitation.

Part 12
Cardiac Trauma

98 A Bullet in Right Ventricle

Joel M. Felner[1] & Jing Ping Sun[2]

[1]Grady Memorial Hospital; Emory University School of Medicine, Atlanta, GA, USA
[2]Emory University School of Medicine; Emory University Hospital Midtown, Atlanta, GA, USA

History

A 20-year-old male was shot at close range during an argument. The assailant employed a 0.22 caliber pistol. A single shot was fired. It penetrated the patient's left anterior thorax and did not exit. His friends rushed him to the hospital within 10 minutes of shooting. The patient was unconscious.

Physical Examination

Blood pressure was 64/40 mmHg; heart rate was 146 bpm; respiratory rate was 24/minute; temperature was 37.2°C. His skin was cold and clammy. An entering wound was noted in the 4th intercostal space just lateral to the mid ventricular area.

The cardiac vascular examination was normal except for rapid heart rate and muffled heart sounds.

The lung exam showed decreased breath sounds bilaterally. Ulterior pulses were weak throughout.

Chest X-ray showed a bullet fragment within the confines of the heart shadow but was unable to document an intracardiac localization.

Echocardiography

Transthoracic echocardiography (TTE) revealed: A diffused unattached echo densed artifact was observed in right ventricular cavity in apical 4-chamber view (Figure 98.1 and Videoclip 98.1)

Treatment

The patient was started on lactated ringers and the blood pressure improved to 100/70 mmHg and the heart rate decreased to 130 bpm.

The patient underwent emergency thoracotomy.

The bullet had lacerated the left anterior pleural into the media sternum and penetrated the pericardial ventricular myocardium. Precise

Practical Handbook of Echocardiography 1st edition. Edited by Jing Ping Sun, Joel Felner and John Merlino. © 2010 Blackwell Publishing Ltd.

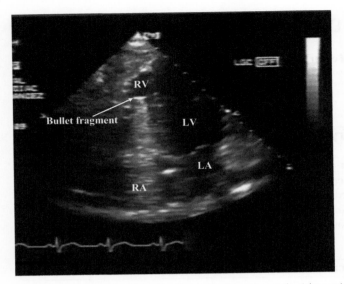

Figure 98.1. A bullet fragment with echo shadow is well seen in the right ventricle. LA, left atrium; LV, left ventricle; RA, right atrium; RV, right ventricle;

localization was not achieved. There was no exit wound. The surgeon elected to oversew the cardiac entry wound rather than extract the bullet.

Post operation, transesophageal echocardiography (TEE) was performed with no change from the preoperative study. The bullet fragment could still be located.

Discussion

Transthoracic echocardiography is capable of confirming the presence or absence of a pericardial effusion. Occasionally the ability to obtain a quality echo study in patients with penetrating cardiac trauma maybe difficult due to chest wall trauma or bandages. In this case, TTE was able to locate the bullet fragment. The echo dense artifact from the bullet fragment was very clear. It is important to localize and characterize intracardiac bullet fragment for the surgeon contemplating a surgery. If TTE is unsuccessful, TEE should be performed to locate and characterize the bullet fragment as well as the extent of myocardial damage.

The characters produced by these metallic objects are of diagnostic value in patients with penetrating missile injuries.

99 Ventricular Septal Defect and Mitral Valve Chordae Transected by Chest Stab

Joel M. Felner[1] & Jing Ping Sun[2]

[1]Grady Memorial Hospital; Emory University School of Medicine, Atlanta, GA, USA
[2]Emory University School of Medicine; Emory University Hospital Midtown, Atlanta, GA, USA

History

A 40-year-old male was conscious after a cardiac stabbing injury when he was brought to the emergence room. A fast study revealed a large pericardial effusion with cardiac tamponade. Central venous pressure was 20 cm of H_2O.

Laboratory Study

Transthoracic echocardiography (TTE) showed a large pericardial effusion with collapse of right atrium and right ventricle (RV) walls. The inferior vena cava was dilated and barely moved with inspiration. Pulse wave Doppler inflow velocities across the mitral valve varied significantly with inspiration. The ratio of systematic to pulmonary blood flow (Qs:Qp) was 1.0:1.8.

Color Doppler echo in the parasternal view demonstrated a ventricular septal defect (VSD) with the pressure gradient to be 71 mmHg.

Transesophageal echocardiography (TEE) was performed after the patient stabilized hemodynamically and demonstrated: (1) VSD at the junction of the middle and lower portion of the intra-ventricular septum with 0.4–0.5 mm in diameter (Figure 99.1), with a significant left to right shunt (Figure 99.1, Videoclip 99.1), (2) posterior papillary muscle proximal mitral valve chordae was transected (Figure 99.2, Videoclip 99.2).

Hospital course: Saline was infused, a chest tube was placed and 800 cc of bloody fluid was drained from the pleural cavity. A subxyphoid pericardiocentesis was performed after the TTE and 300 cc of bloody fluid was removed. A median sternotomy was performed and a 2.5-cm stab wound to the RV was oversewn.

At surgery, the cardiac defect measured up to 1.4 cm in diameter. It ran obliquely through the intraventricular septum and one proximal mitral

Practical Handbook of Echocardiography 1st edition. Edited by Jing Ping Sun, Joel Felner and John Merlino. © 2010 Blackwell Publishing Ltd.

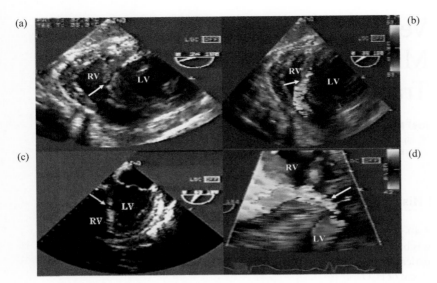

Figure 99.1. Transesophageal echocardiogram images show a defect (arrows) located on the basal segment of the ventricular septum (a and c). A hemodynamically significant ventricular septal defect with a left to right shunt was present (arrows, b and d). LV, left ventricle; RV, right ventricle.

valve chordae was transected. The VSD was closed with a patch and mitral valve replacement was performed with a St. Jude number 29 prosthesis. Intraoperative TEE excluded any residual shunt. The postoperation course was uneventful and the patient was discharged on postoperative day 6.

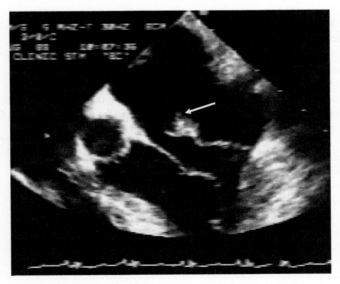

Figure 99.2. Transesophageal echocardiography showed that one proximal mitral valve chordaewas transected (arrow).

Discussion

Trauma represents the third most common cause of death in the USA after cancer and cardiovascular disease. All penetrating wounds that appear to involve the heart must be diagnosed quickly because accumulation of blood within the pericardium causes cardiac tamponade and hemodynamic decompensation.

The most frequent cause of penetrating trauma to the heart is a stab injury. The RV is injured in about half of surviving patients and LV less often. About 25% of the patients are diagnosed as having a VSD caused by penetrating injury to the heart. In most cases a stab injury to the heart leads to cardiac tamponade.

A fast study is the diagnostic test of choice for the initial evaluation of patients with penetrating precordial injury. Echocardiography is the gold standard in the evaluation of patients with penetrating thoracic injury [1].

If the patient is stable after the initial evaluation, a complete TTE should be performed within 6 hours to improve diagnostic accuracy. If this cannot be accomplished, a TEE should be done.

Aggressive management, including cardiorrhaphy when indicated, is currently recognized to lead to more optimal results than conservative management [2].

References

1. Jimenez E, Martin M, Krukenkamp I, *et al.* Subxiphoid pericardiotomy versus echocardiography: a prospective evaluation of the diagnosis of occult penetrating cardiac injury. *Surgery* 1990;108:676–80.
2. Sugg WL, Rea WJ, Ecker RR, *et al.* Penetrating wounds of the heart: an analysis of 459 cases. *J Thorac Cardiovasc Surg* 1968;56:531–45.

100 Aorta-Right Ventricular Fistula Caused by Chest Stab

Joel M. Felner[1] & Jing Ping Sun[2]

[1]Grady Memorial Hospital; Emory University School of Medicine, Atlanta, GA, USA
[2]Emory University School of Medicine; Emory University Hospital Midtown, Atlanta, GA, USA

History

A 30-year-old male complains of shortness of breath and chest pain as he sustained a knife wound in the left anterior chest about 15 minutes ago.

Physical Examination

A 2.6-cm wound was located approximately 2.4 cm lateral to the left nipple. Blood pressure was 104/82 mmHg; pulse rate was 106/minute and respiratory rate was 22/minute. Lung exam: decreased breath sounds on the left side with no evidence of a sucking chest wound. Cardiac examination: There was a grade 3/6 systolic murmur.

Laboratory

Chest X-ray revealed a large left pleural effusion and an enlarged cardiopericardial silhouette.

Transthoracic echocardiography (TTE) revealed normal chamber sizes and normal ventricular systolic function. There was a moderate amount of pericardial fluid but no evidence of cardiac tamponade.

Transesophageal echocardiography (TEE) showed a 2 mm area of echo dropout in the ascending aorta located approximately 3 mm lateral to the origin of the right coronary artery. Color Doppler echo revealed a jet traversed through the wall of the ascending aorta into the right ventricle (Figure 100.1, and Videoclip 100.1)

Hospital Course

This defect was oversewn with a pericardial patch during cardiopulmonary bypass. The patient was discharged in stable condition 9 days after operation.

Practical Handbook of Echocardiography 1st edition. Edited by Jing Ping Sun, Joel Felner and John Merlino. © 2010 Blackwell Publishing Ltd.

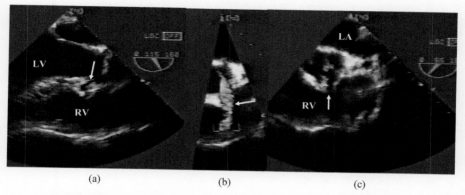

(a)   (b)   (c)

Figure 100.1. Transthoracic echocardiography revealed a 2-mm area of echo dropout (arrow) in the ascending aorta located approximately 3 mm lateral to the origin of right coronary artery (a). Color Doppler showed flow across an aorta–right ventricle (arrow) just distal to right coronary artery (b). The short axis of aorta showed a 2-mm area of echo dropout (arrow) in the ascending aorta (c). LA, left atrium; LV, left ventricle; RV, right ventricle.

Discussion

Even after penetrating cardiac injury a shunt is not always immediately created. A fistula may be created or enlarged over time in an area of weakness. As in our case, discovery of a defect can be delayed days after the initial insult. A murmur is usually appreciated, however.

The best approach to evaluating these patients is to utilize serial echocardiography. Two-dimensional echo has been found to be 90% sensitive and 97% specific for the diagnoses of cardiac penetration [1]. Echocardiography can rapidly establish the diagnoses in patients with various forms of trauma. The FAST (focused assessment with sonography in trauma) study is both sensitive and specific into the determination of traumatic pericardial effusion and intraperitoneal fluid indicative of injury thus effectively guiding emergency surgical decision making [2]. In addition a complete TTE should be performed. However, a complete TTE does not always identify intracardiac lesions even with technically adequate study. TEE is especially beneficial in the severely hemodynamically compromised trauma patient in the acute setting and in the immediate recovery phase.

The most important factor for survival is rapid diagnoses and immediate treatment. Most of these patients need emergency thoracotomy to relieve tamponade. Suspicion of intracardiac injury is usually raised by persistent hemodynamic instability or the incidental discovery of a cardiac murmur. Many of these lesions maybe come clinically detectable only at a later stage when the defect will become larger after resolution of the surrounding edema. Depending upon the injury there may be a delay of several days between the initial insult and evidence of injury.

References

1. Jimenez E, Martin M, Krukenkamp I, Barrett J. Subxiphoid pericardiotomy versus echocardiography: a prospective evaluation of the diagnosis of occult penetrating cardiac injury. *Surgery* 1990; 108(4): 676–80.
2. Tayal VS, Beatty MA, Marx JA, Tomaszewski CA, Thomason MH. FAST (Focused Assessment With Sonography in Trauma) accurate for cardiac and intraperitoneal injury in penetrating anterior chest trauma. *J Ultrasound Med* 2004;23(4): 467–72.

101 A Nail in Aorta

Joel M. Felner[1] & Jing Ping Sun[2]

[1]Grady Memorial Hospital; Emory University School of Medicine, Atlanta, GA, USA
[2]Emory University School of Medicine; Emory University Hospital Midtown, Atlanta, GA, USA

History

A 50-year-old depressed man shot himself in the chest with a nail gun. He presented to the emergency room in shock and short of breath.

Physical Examination

Blood pressure was 90/60, heart rate was 120 with paradox pulse, respiration rate was 28, and temperature was normal. Neck veins were distended. Carotid pulses were weak. Apex impulse was not palpable. No audible murmurs or gallops.

Laboratory

Electrocardiogram showed the presence of sinus tachycardia, otherwise within normal limits. Chest X-ray: large cardio-pericardial silhouette with pulmonary congestion. Nail could be seen in the middle of the heart. Transthoracic echocardiography: difficult to perform; small pericardial effusion was detected.

Treatment

Emergency surgery with transesophageal echocardiography (TEE) guidance was conducted. TEE revealed a nail in the aorta just distal to aortic leaflets and <1 cm distal to the right coronary artery (Figure 101.1, Videoclip 101.1). It missed the pulmonic valve as it penetrated through the right ventricle. It allowed the surgeon to locate the nail, which was not initially seen when the chest was opened. The surgeon successfully removed the nail and 500 cc of bloody fluid without incident. A psychiatric consultation revealed that his girlfriend had broke up with him that morning. He was discharged without further incident in 7 days with follow-up of psychiatry and surgery.

Practical Handbook of Echocardiography 1st edition. Edited by Jing Ping Sun, Joel Felner and John Merlino. © 2010 Blackwell Publishing Ltd.

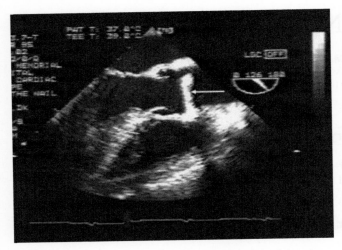

Figure 101.1. A nail is clearly seen by transesophageal echocardiogram image.

Discussion

This case is a rare cardiac trauma; echocardiography is a useful diagnosis tool to locate the penetrate material.

Index

Printed and bound by CPI Group (UK) Ltd, Croydon, CR0 4YY

16/04/2025

14658826-0001